Everything I l

Also by Sujay Kansagra

Vault's Medical School Admissions

EVERYTHING
I LEARNED IN
MEDICAL SCHOOL
Besides All the Book Stuff

By

Sujay M. Kansagra, MD

To Mom, Dad, Susan, Shayri,
Rajesh, Neil, and Baa,
for their everlasting support.
And to my wife, Sejal, who
has voluntarily agreed to
spend her life with me. I'm still
not sure why.

Author's Note

These stories are all true. Where appropriate, names have been changed to protect the identities of patients, physicians, and medical students.

Contents

Preface

This book began as something much different. In the beginning, it was something just for me. It was a way to remember how it felt to walk into my first patient's room, to relive the exhilaration of delivering my first baby, and to remember the frustration of being lost in a world with an entirely new language. I wanted to look back after becoming old and gray, and remember how the world of medicine looked to someone seeing it with fresh eyes. These eyes were free from years of becoming jaded and were filled with curiosity, excitement, and nervous anticipation. But as this work took shape, I began to realize it could be more. It could be a way to show others this strange new world and to share the lessons I learned along the way that applied not only to medicine, but to everyday life. And through this journey, I came across those patients and doctors that were just so entertaining, so over the top, they were almost asking for their stories to be told. This is my way of sharing those stories. So here I am, giving you a glimpse into a life of medicine as I first saw it during medical school.

Please do not mistake some of the jokes and criticisms of medicine in this book for cynicism. Not a day went by during medical school that I did not feel grateful to be a part of medicine, to have the privilege of hearing about intimate aspects of people's lives, and to help them through their most difficult times. And at the same time, there are situations where it's okay to laugh at ourselves, laugh with our patients, and laugh at the insanity that surrounds us on a daily basis in the hospital. It keeps us grounded. So here it is, my four years of medical school -- the serious, the stressful, the funny, the unbelievable, the unexplainable, the sick, the struggles, and the stories that taught me everything I learned in medical school (besides all the book stuff, of course).

Chapter 1

That Sinking Feeling

My body jolts awake to a familiar sound. After a few blind swipes, my blows hit their target, and once again, there is silence. The air in the room is cool, crisp, and every fiber of my being wants me to remain in the welcoming warmth under the covers. It is Saturday morning, and any other Saturday of my life I would be waking only when my body was ready. But this month was different. My body no longer called the shots.

I clumsily make my way around, grab my towel and clothes, and walk out of the room, squinting at the bright lights in the living room. My roommate, still up playing video games, looks at me, then his watch, then back at me.

"Wow, one of us is pretty pathetic."

"I think we both are," I reply.

It is 3AM. As a second year medical student, rotations have taken over my life. This particular month happens to be dedicated to pediatric surgery, one of the many fields through which I would rotate this year. I'm quickly learning that the popular notion that medical students are sleep deprived is popular for a reason. I'm also beginning to realize that life's priorities have a funny way of coming full circle. When you're first born, your main priority in life is sleeping. When you're nine, the priorities are Saturday morning cartoons and baseball cards. In college, it's staying out late and partying. But in medical school, your priorities go back to the beginning -- sleeping. This becomes more evident the longer you are on the wards.

Imagine falling into a pool filled with caramel. You try desperately to swim out, but you slowly sink to the bottom, and there you are, looking up to see a brown-tinged world. Despite all of your best efforts to swim out, the caramel is just too thick. You barely get halfway to the top before you give up, and defeated, find yourself sinking back down to the bottom. This is how it feels when the sleep deprivation starts kicking in. There is a constant fog over you. The minute you sit down to relax or for a lecture, it starts. You become one with your chair, as you feel yourself settling in. Your eyelids feel like they are attached to lead weights. Your body goes into shutdown mode, and slowly but surely, you start sinking into the caramel pool. There is nothing you can do to swim out of it. I've tried it all. Caffeine was of little use. A few times, I tried pinching my leg as hard as possible when no one was looking. It helps for about 30 seconds, and then I'm back to where I started. One time I tried asking a question during a lecture to force myself to wake up and pay attention, only to have the lecturer reply that she had been answering that very question for the last ten minutes of the lecture, making me look very foolish. That worked at getting me awake, but at a price.

The sleep factor plays a larger role during some rotations more than others, namely, Internal Medicine and Surgery. Shifts in excess of thirty straight hours are commonplace for residents in these fields. Despite regulations which mandate a maximum of 80 hours of work per week, logging false duty hours and working over 100 hours is not unheard of. It is all part of the "suck it up" mentality that runs rampant and unchecked in medicine. I'm convinced that the interview process for these two fields involves keeping applicants awake for 48 hours and then asking them to do Calculus. It's just unreal.   During this pediatric surgery rotation, I finally reached the end of my rope.

We spent a good deal of time in the operating room during this month. For a medical student in the operating room, our job consists solely of three things: cutting, holding, and suctioning. We cut suture when the surgeon is finished tying, we hold back flaps of skin with equipment called retractors, and we suction fluid and blood using a small vacuum tube. After days and days of waking up early, this can get a bit boring. Well, on one particular day, it was 9AM, and we had already seen two surgery cases. This was the third. The case was a simple inguinal hernia repair, so unfortunately, there was no suctioning, cutting, or retracting to be had, so I stood there, with arms crossed in front of me, so as not to touch something accidentally and contaminate the entire surgery. About ten minutes into the case, I could feel the sweet voice of sleep calling my name, but I hung on. The case continued, as they operated on a very small area that I could barely even see. My mind began to wander, as I thought of how nice it would be if I were anywhere else. The image of my room and my warm bed arose, almost like an oasis for a bone-dry wanderer through the desert. And just then, out of nowhere, my body felt a unique sensation. It was a numbness that went through me, and was followed by the sensation of falling. But just then, I felt my body jerk, and as quickly as it had started, the numbness and falling sensation stopped. For the first time in my life, I had fallen asleep standing up! But not long enough to fall over, just enough to jerk to one side and catch myself, not unlike the head jerks you see people doing in the classroom. Except this was a full body jerk. Luckily, the movement was subtle enough that no one noticed. I guess they were too busy operating.

After this, the sleep-while-standing incidents (which I call "steeping") were happening on a regular basis in the OR. During just about every surgery, I would have the now familiar sensation of falling and quickly jerking awake. Even if there was a retractor in my hand, I slowly faded out, and the tension on the retractor would slowly give way, only to be awoken by the surgeon grabbing the retractor and repositioning it. But, despite this, no one noticed that I was actually falling "asteep", not even the nurse that would hand the surgeon the various instruments. On one occasion, I actually fell towards the surgeon and bumped him while he was operating. Luckily, the senior resident had the scalpel at the time, and I disguised my bump as an effort to get a better look at the surgery. That was a close one. Thankfully, this was near the end of my rotation, and there was never a serious incident.

The battles with sleep are not unfamiliar to medical students. One of my fellow students was standing at the foot of a patient's bed while the entire medical team was in the room talking with the patient. This 6'4" guy fell asleep and landed directly on the patient! Luckily, there were no injuries, except perhaps to the student's grade (and pride). I quickly learned that sleep cannot be cheated; it always gets its just due, one way or another.

Hopefully, when I finish all of my training and become an attending physician, the priorities will shift back in the cartoon direction. But the huge pool of caramel known as residency is around the corner, and there are no life guards on duty.

Chapter 2

The Switcheroo

Nothing was out of the ordinary as my morning began. The holding area that led to the operating rooms was abuzz. The place exuded that hospital feel, with white walls, white floors, and the smell of various antiseptic cleaning concoctions. Everyone walking around was wearing little blue shoe covers and matching blue hair covers, the type of stuff you see surgeons wearing that make them look like they belong. There were anesthesiologists standing next to patients on stretchers, explaining how they would be put to sleep for their procedures. There were ophthalmologists walking around, getting ready for their next cases or casually chatting with fellow eye doctors. And there I was, the lone medical student, trying to find an interesting surgery to go see. Little did I know that this morning, I would run into the most peculiar patient I had ever seen.

It was my fourth and final year of medical school, and this was my ophthalmology rotation. The entire surgical suite was dedicated to eye surgery. For the entire month, I would follow various doctors and simply watch as they performed intricate surgeries. Frankly, things were getting dull. I had already seen enough cataract surgeries to last me a lifetime. But on the schedule for that day was a case I had not seen before. When the case was about to begin, I walked into the operating room, mask on my face, ready to see something new.

The resident was already in the operating room. He saw me walk in and gave me a quick overview of the patient.

"He's had an inflammatory reaction in the upper cheeks, bilaterally," he said, very matter-of-factly. "We've got to go in there and break things up a little, because the inflammation has tightened up his cheeks to the point he can't close his eyes."

One glance over at the sedated patient on the operating table and I knew something didn't quite fit. The resident kept making reference to "he" and "his". Yet the patient clearly had the facial features of a female. High cheekbones. No facial hair in sight. Maybe the resident was just mistaken.

The nurses began performing the mandatory "time out". This is a safety precaution in which they verify that the patient is indeed the proper patient, and the procedure is the appropriate procedure. As you can imagine, one of the biggest mistakes you can make as a surgeon is operating on the wrong person, performing the wrong operation, or operating on the wrong side, so this part is critical. But even the nurse performing the timeout began with, "*He* is here for bilateral…"

The resident must have seen my confused glances at the patient, so he kindly filled me in. The patient was indeed a male, but with transgender identity disorder. Simply put, he wanted to be a female. So, in order to look more like a female, he had gotten laser surgery on all of his facial hair. In addition, this patient had gotten silicone injections in his buttocks, lips and cheeks. It was the silicone injections in his cheeks that had gone horribly wrong, and the reason he was on the operating table that day.

It was one year earlier when the patient checked into a hotel to participate in a "silicone party". This was a party in which two guys would inject silicone into whatever body part a participant desired. For their services, they charged a small fee. Unfortunately, these two "plastic surgeons" were not doctors at all, just some guys looking to make a few quick bucks. Many questions are probably going through your head at this point. Why would someone go to a hotel for this procedure? Why would you trust random people to inject a foreign material into your body if you knew they weren't doctors? What was this person thinking?! All good questions. I have no answers for you.

To make matters worse, the silicone these pseudo-surgeons were injecting was not exactly medical grade silicone. In fact, it was purchased from a local Home Depot®. It doesn't take a medical professional to realize that this is bad news. For this patient, the lip and buttock injections worked just fine. However, the cheeks had developed an inflammatory reaction to the silicone. It was his body's way of saying, "Tiss, tiss, tiss." Apparently, this silicone wasn't meant for direct human injection. Go figure. The ophthalmologist had to dig under the inside of his upper lip, go under both cheeks and up to his eye socket to implant a device to hold his cheeks up. This would allow him to actually shut his eyes. Not the result this patient probably had in mind when signing up for the silicone party.

It is hard to imagine what drives people in their daily decisions. At what point does having an untrained man in a hotel inject silicone into your body seem like an acceptable decision? But then again, we're all guilty of making choices that others would think were crazy. I decided to go to medical school, which some would consider crazy. Some people decide to smoke. Others may consider driving a motorcycle crazy. It all depends on where we set our "crazy meter". But when it comes to plastic surgery, everyone should sound their "crazy alarm" at a low setting.

And in case you're wondering, the rogue, silicone-injecting "plastic surgeons" are now serving a prison sentence.

Chapter 3

The Hierarchy

Imagine an ordinary place of work. Let's say it's an office building for an investment banking firm. There are two people standing at the water cooler. One is a mere associate, while the other is the vice-president of the company. Just by looking, it is often hard to tell which is which. Now, let's pretend we're walking around in the hospital. Here, figuring out who's the boss is not so difficult. Imagine that the boss (aka, the attending doctor) now has a cape with fluorescent colors that indicate his superior rank. Along with this is a hat with flashing lights that not so discretely spell out, "I'm your daddy". And in case you missed both of these, he or she has an entourage of residents and interns that fan him and feed him grapes.

Okay, it may be a little more subtle than this, but it's obvious that in the hospital, the hierarchy is everywhere, and it's in your face constantly. For starters, those that are higher ranking have longer coats. Most attendings have white coats that reach their knees. A slightly shorter coat goes to the resident, who is still in training, but far enough out from medical school that they know what they are doing. An even smaller coat is worn by the intern, the title given to an MD during their first year after completing medical school. And no, they don't know what they're doing. And then there's the medical student, whose coat resembles a tight fitting, full-sleeved vest, the kind that makes your arms pull away from your body. In addition to coat length, every doctor has their name clearly written on their coat, along with every degree they've ever received. Every now and then, I'll spot an MD, JD, MPH. If this isn't enough hierarching (which must be a word), the doctor's field of expertise is clearly written below the name, which adds yet another level of superiority to those lucky enough to be neurosurgeons and cardiologists.

The totem pole carries over in even the most subtle of actions in the hospital. For example, watching a team of attendings, residents, interns and medical students walk around the hospital is an easy way to quickly decipher who's who (in case the coat length, embroidered letters indicating degree, and flashing hat weren't enough). The

13

key is paying attention to the order in which they walk. For those of you interested in medical school, I've taken it upon myself to help teach you this order. Below you will find appropriate walking orders. Just for clarification purposes, "1" indicates the person in the lead, "2" is second, and so forth. More than one person next to the number indicates people walking side-by-side. Here we go...

Acceptable walking order:
1. Attending, senior resident
2. Intern
3. Medical students

or...
1. Attending
2. Senior Resident, Intern
3. Medical students

or even...
1. Attending, senior resident
2. Intern, medical student (the kiss up one)
3. Medical student (the nervous one)

The following are unacceptable, and rarely ever seen:
1. Attending physician, intern
2. Senior resident, medical students

or...

1. Intern
2. Attending, medical students
3. Resident

and definitely, definitely not...

1. Medical student
2. Anyone else

Another situation in which the hierarchy becomes obvious is when an attending tells a joke. First and foremost, if someone on the team tells a joke, you can pretty much say with certainty that this person is the attending. No one else would dare attempt to add humor to the workday. Every so often, the joke will actually be funny, in which case everyone laughs briefly and moves on, not allowing us to determine the rest of the hierarchy. But 9 times out of 10, the joke is not so funny, and that's when, once again, rank becomes obvious. First, everyone must laugh, it's required. So, residents, interns, and medical students all begin. The fake laugh in and of itself is hard to master, since it's usually pretty easy to see through a fake laugh, so this must be practiced. So there is the team, laughing away. Pretty soon, the resident stops laughing, and taking the cue from the resident, the intern soon stops as well. If there is only one medical student, they can stop laughing soon after the intern and life is good. But if there is more than one medical student around, this part starts getting tricky. Each student feels they have to be the last medical student laughing so as to show the attending they thought the joke was funnier than their fellow medical student, thereby obtaining the favor of the attending, and a better evaluation at the end. Unfortunately, at some point, the laughing goes on for so long that it becomes obvious you are faking it. So, for two dueling medical students, it all comes down to who can laugh the longest, but stop right at the time it starts looking fake. This is challenging. Many factors play into how long you can carry on the laugh, such as how convincing you can be (an occasional knee slap never hurts, but more than one knee slap is pushing it), how gullible the attending is (does he actually believe he's funny?), and the jaded level of the resident (the more jaded, the shorter time the student should laugh, so as not to make residents mad for prolonging the torture of rounds). The combination that worked well for me was a simple head throw (where I throw my head back and laugh into the air for a few seconds), followed by a few head nods as the laughing dies down, and finished off with a, "that's too funny."

Hopefully these little walking and laughing lessons will help you easily figure out who's who in the hospital, not to mention provide useful tips to those aspiring to be physicians. You can thank me later.

But in all seriousness, there has to be a reason that such a hierarchy is so entrenched in the medical world. Is it because it makes it easier for patients to identify the head physicians? Doubt it. Is it because after years of studying and working, doctors feel entitled to some recognition? Possibly. Does it just feel good to be the boss after years of getting bullied as a kid for being the smart one? Probably. But as it turns out, not every attending physician behaves like royalty. In fact, quite a few treat residents as equals, are very approachable for medical students, and seem to really enjoy their work. One soon realizes that the hierarchy-loving, order-spouting attendings often hide behind their rank. Perhaps they are not as comfortable with their knowledge or skills as a physician, causing anxiety which translates into emphasizing their rank on the medical totem pole. So, look for those doctors that walk in the back of the pack, don't mind when you don't laugh at their jokes, talk to nurses with respect, say hello to the janitors, and don't worry about rank. I've learned that they are the smart ones.

Chapter 4

I Don't Even Know You Anymore

History has molded our impression of medicine into that of a noble field. With rare exception, doctors throughout the world are held in high regards. After all, they are deemed to be intelligent, hard working, ethical people, who have dedicated their lives to the welfare of others. They are role models for a healthy lifestyle. We start to believe all of these lies very early in life.

As a child, my parents and I made frequent trips to the pediatrician for my mild asthma problem. There were multiple doctors in this practice, and it never really mattered to me which one I saw. After all, every doctor was smart, capable, and knew exactly what to do. They seemed incredibly honest, trustworthy and confident, making it easy for my parents to place the burden of handling my health concerns on them. Whatever the doctor said, we would do. They seemed like perfect people, with all the answers.

Medical school quickly changed my perception of doctors. The first blow was during a party to celebrate the half-way mark through our first year. We had completed many of our basic science courses, which included anatomy, genetics, physiology and biochemistry. During this time, we had dissected the lungs of cancer patients and learned about the cellular mechanisms that can go awry on the way to developing cancer. There were detailed discussions on genetic predispositions to this terrible disease, and how its risk was multiplied significantly by exposure to compounds such as cigarette smoke. If I hadn't already decided, these lectures were enough to convince me to stay miles away from cigarettes. Not only that, I was prepared to help stamp out the "cancer stick" amongst my future patients. But despite these lectures and this knowledge, I was surprised to see a group of future doctors proudly puffing away at this party. Somewhere in my brain was a small part that refused to believe doctors, or future doctors, would do this kind of thing, the same way that I refused to believe movie stars had to poop when

I was a little kid. These people couldn't possibly do something so disgusting. And yet I was seeing it first hand (the smoking, that is).

But this was only the beginning. Over the years, there were countless stories of other questionable behaviors that I could not imagine my doctors doing as medical students. Anything from multiple classmates using marijuana, to snorting prescription pain medications, to alcohol abuse, and even close associations with exotic dancers, we had it all. There were stories of debauchery between students and our superiors, unstable cases of depression and anxiety, as well as, trouble with the law. The revelation that these future physicians were far from perfect with their own health and well-being was frightening. How would we hold our patients to a higher standard when we couldn't even manage our own health?

But then again, perhaps the mold that doctors are expected to fit is a bit unfair. Does it matter what vices a physician deals with so long as it does not impact patient care? I must admit, I did not figure out an answer to this. What I did learn is that doctors and future doctors have the same problems everyone else does. Going to medical school doesn't grant you a "get-out-of-problems-free" card. Having in-depth knowledge about the risks of smoking and drugs does not shield you from their allure. Because as it turns out, everyone poops.

Chapter 5

The Pressure's On

Halfway through medical school, life as a student takes an abrupt turn. In most medical schools, the first two years consist of sitting in a large, rather unstimulating classroom, hearing lectures for hours on end. Some pay attention, while others chat online or daydream. For the most part, it's a rather comfortable, undemanding environment. But as the third year of medical school starts (or in our case, the second year), we're suddenly plucked out of our classroom seats that have become so cozy, and dropped into a whole new world. This is when we start learning in a different environment -- inside the hospital. Our medical school had only one year of classroom lectures, and we spent our second and fourth years working in the hospital. The third year we will talk about later. So, one year into medical school, we are thrown into the thick of it. Most of our time is spent on the inpatient side of the hospital (aka, the wards) as opposed to working in clinics where people come in for regular appointments. Here is how the wards work… students are assigned to a particular field of medicine for one or two months, such as pediatrics, internal medicine, surgery, obstetrics and gynecology, etc. Each of these fields has a number of teams, and each team consists of an attending, resident, a few interns, and the patients they take care of. As a medical student, you are part of a particular team and follow two to three patients. You aren't truly taking care of them, but it's mostly a way to pretend you are, in order to learn how medicine is practiced. The typical day consists of the students, interns, and residents getting there early, seeing all of the patients and collecting information from overnight, such as whether the patient had a fever, laboratory results, interpretation of x-rays, etc. Then, later in the morning, the attending shows up and the entire team goes from patients' room to room (or sits down in a conference room) and talks about all the patients. This is known as "rounds".

Any student that has been through rounds for the first time can tell you this is when it becomes blatantly clear that the comfortable days of sinking into your classroom chair and daydreaming are very much over. You are now constantly asked to perform in front of a crowd of doctors. When it's time to talk about your patient, you discuss how the patient did overnight, how the patient feels that morning, vital signs, new lab results, physical exam, and a plan for the day. It sounds fairly straightforward, but when you're in front of the entire team, it's not that easy. Plus, this is one of the few times a student actually interacts with the attending physician, so your grade is often influenced by how calmly, comfortably, and succinctly you can give the presentation.

I consider myself a pretty calm guy. Public speaking was never really a problem for me, and I felt comfortable in front of a crowd. But this was a totally different feeling. Not only are you in front of a crowd, but this crowd knows a lot more than you do about your topic. I think of it as trying to give a physics presentation in front of Einstein or Stephen Hawking. Well, maybe not that bad, but you get the point. So, one Saturday during my surgery rotation, I was rounding with the team. So far, I had been incredibly composed during rounds. But today, the senior resident made it a point to say we were going to try to move fast through the patients so we could get home. After all, it was the weekend. No problem, I thought to myself, I'll present my patients quickly and succinctly.

We were walking around fast, from room to room. My patients were coming up, and I felt the rush of nervousness, knowing I had to impress the team. We rushed up and down flights of stairs to get to patients on other floors. My heart started racing and I was a little out of breath from all the moving around. And before I knew it, we were at the door of my first patient. I started the presentation, and it came out in chunks in between the breaths I was taking. There was this feeling of discomfort, as if my heart was beating so hard that it was pressing against my wind pipe. I tried to go on with the presentation as if I was merely catching my breath, but it soon became obvious to me, and to the team, that there was more going on. "Man, I can't catch my breath," I said, trying to hide my obvious discomfort. "Calm down, you're doing fine," the resident said, not fooled by my cover-up. I couldn't believe it, this had never happened to me before. I was hyperventilating! "Oh, no, I'm just short of breath," I said, trying to save face. Eventually calming down, I proceeded with the rest of the presentation. As we walked around that morning, I occasionally threw in comments on how out of shape I was, hoping the team would buy it. But

I think we all knew what had happened. How embarrassing.

The presentation itself can be tough, but there is yet another part of rounding that can increase sphincter tone, and that's having the whole team go in and talk with the patient. You've just stood outside the door with the entire team telling them how the patient is doing that morning, and everything you thought was relevant. Then, you pray that the patient doesn't say something contradictory, making you look like a liar, or add something new to the story, making you look incompetent. It's probably not that difficult to believe that the patient's story changes all the time. For example, the patient tells you they are having sharp, stabbing belly pain, which you tell the team, but when you go in the room and ask the patient, they say it is dull, crushing chest pain. The student stands there, turning slightly red, wanting to cry out, "BUT YOU TOLD ME EARLIER THAT...," but usually the doctor just keeps talking without even giving the student a look. Meanwhile, the student is wondering whether the doctor even caught on to the discrepancy, and if they are going to mention it after walking out of the room. Nine times out of ten, the doctor doesn't mention anything, either because they expect students to mess up, because they know that the patient's story changes all the time, or the most likely reason, they weren't listening to the student's presentation in the first place.

One of the more entertaining presentation experiences happened to a fellow medical student while on the neurology service. On this rotation, students are expected to do neurologic physical exams on patients in the morning to assess if there are any changes. The majority of patients on the neurology service have had strokes, so any changes in the exam, like new areas of weakness, could indicate a worsening stroke. This exam includes a "Cranial Nerve" exam, which tests the important nerves of the head, neck and shoulders. These are the nerves that are important in sight, taste, touch, hearing, movement, etc. The second cranial nerve is called the optic nerve, and it is responsible for vision. To test a patient's peripheral vision, an examiner will often have the patient stare straight ahead and have them report how many fingers the examiner is holding up on the sides. Likewise, there are ways to test the function of the other cranial nerves. When the entire cranial nerve exam is finished, and if everything is normal, doctors typically report, "Cranial Nerves 2 through 12 are intact." Cranial nerve 1 is the olfactory nerve, responsible for smell, which we don't typically check unless the patient complains about problems smelling. So, on rounds, it's typical for a student to start the physical exam presentation by stating, "For the neuro exam, cranial nerves 2 through 12 are intact." Well, this particular day was the student's first day on the rotation, and he had to pick up patients that had been in the hospital for a few days. So, the other members of the team were already familiar with the patients. That morning, the student had rounded on his patients bright and early. When rounding began with the team, they eventually got to his patient and stood outside of the room to discuss the case. So, he began his presentation. When he got to the physical exam portion, he calmly told the team,

"Cranial Nerves 2 through 12 intact."

Before he could go on with the rest of his exam findings, the attending interrupted, "What did you say?"

"Cranial Nerves 2 through 12 intact," the student repeated, this time somewhat more hesitant.

"That's not possible," the resident said.

The student stood there, confused at where he went wrong. The attending, at this point somewhat perturbed, asked,

"Did you actually go in to examine this patient?"

"Yes, of course."

"Well, his cranial nerves can't all be intact, because the patient is blind!"

The student looked shocked at this, and explained to the team that he even tested his peripheral vision, and everything seemed fine. So, the team walked into the room, intent on resolving the two discrepant stories. The attending went up to the patient, and asked simply,

"Sir, can you see my hand waving in front of you?"

"No, I've been blind for years."

At this point, the student had to speak up.

"But sir, when I came in this morning, and tested your vision, you kept telling me how many fingers I was holding up."

To which the patient calmly replied, "Oh, I was just guessing."

Turns out this patient was a great guesser, and the team ended up having a good laugh.

In any given day, there are multiple pressure-filled situations in the hospital or any other work place that can get you upset or test your composure. Sometimes, you have to take a step back and just laugh at yourself. For a student, it can make the difference between being constantly stressed in a new, challenging environment and truly being able to relax and enjoy the new learning experience.

Chapter 6
"Nursing" Homes

One of the most difficult groups of patients to treat in the hospital are those that come from nursing homes. These are the patients that are either too sick to be cared for at home, or those whose families simply don't have the time to care for. Although one would hope that the money families put into nursing homes would ensure their loved ones are looked after, this sadly is sometimes not the case.

One particular patient stands out vividly. It was during my Internal Medicine rotation that this African American man in his 50s was admitted for worsening of his congestive heart failure (CHF). CHF starts when, for one reason or another, a person's heart isn't able to work well enough to pump blood to their organs. Blood starts backing up in the veins, and fluid begins to leak out because of the pressure. This causes swelling all over, most commonly in the legs. Well, this unfortunate man had swelling in only one leg. His other leg had been amputated long ago from gangrene, which happens when blood stops flowing in an extremity. Despite having a prosthetic leg, he couldn't stand up, because his heart wasn't able to keep up with the stress of pumping blood all the way up to his head against gravity. If he tried to stand, he would pass out. Truly unfortunate. But to make matters worse, his wife no longer wanted him living at home because taking care of him was such a huge burden. You can imagine how difficult it would be to bathe and change a 300 pound man on a daily basis. So he spent his time in a nursing home.

While in the hospital, the team took good care of him. We gave him furosemide, which is a drug that helped him urinate the extra fluid that had built up. We even got him a new prosthetic leg, which fit much better than his old one. He was in remarkably good spirits through all of this, despite his illness. After nearly a week, his swelling had improved, and he was ready to leave the hospital. I walked in early that morning to share the good news.

"You're all set. Looks like you've lost a bunch of that fluid. We should have you back to the nursing home this afternoon."

I was expecting a smile, and a sigh of relief, but he gave me neither.

"Please don't send me back there."

He explained how each morning, he would wake up around 8AM. For the next few hours, he would simply lay there. The staff would argue about whose turn it was to lift him to sit him up. This was all done within earshot. It wasn't until lunch time on most days that he would be helped into a sitting position, where he could finally look out the window, eat, or watch TV. "People just shouldn't be treated like that," he told me. I truly felt sorry for him, wishing we could just keep him in the hospital with us. But as a resident once told me, the hospital is no hotel. Patients have to leave. I told him I would check to see if we could get him into another nursing home, and he was grateful.

So off I went to the social worker's office, with my hopes high. One look at his insurance, and the social worker explained that there was no other place that would accept him. He was stuck. It was truly unfortunate when he had to leave, knowing that he would return to the same miserable conditions, trapped within his own body, unable to care for himself. Each day he would face the same humiliation and inconsiderate disregard by the staff. It was disturbing. It was inhumane.

Later during that month, an old lady in her 80s was admitted, virtually comatose. She was incredibly dehydrated, and looked shriveled up. The lady was slightly demented, and for some reason, she stopped drinking and eating in her nursing home. When she got dehydrated, she started losing consciousness. But that didn't stop the nursing home staff from bringing out her juice bottles with her meals, and watching them pile up on her desk. Apparently, it wasn't their job to make sure she drank them, just so long as she got them. When her daughter arrived to visit a few days later, she was rightfully horrified, and brought her to the hospital. When an elderly person doesn't drink for 2-3 days, the body starts shutting down. To make matters worse, when we went into her room to examine her and turned her to one side, her hip had a bed sore that had torn through her skin and eroded all the way to her hip bone! This is what happens to the skin when someone is bed ridden and unable to change positions (or in this case, when no one helps you change positions). The hole was oozing yellow, foul smelling pus. This was a human being, very much alive, but rotting to death.

All it took were a few bags of saline into her veins, and she was up and talking again, asking for hotdogs and juice. And off she went, back to her nursing home. It would be only a matter of time until she returned again.

This is not to say that all nursing homes are negligent. To the contrary, there are no doubt some that take very good care of their inhabitants. There is also little doubt that the amount these particular homes charge will cause you to have a heart attack and die before you can truly enjoy their services. Either way, I hope that my children continue in the tradition that is a big part of my culture. That is, to have the parents take care of the children while they are young, and then the children take care of the parents when they get old. It's a beautiful system, because in the end, when you're old and gray, if your family won't look after you, I learned it's hard to count on anyone else.

Chapter 7

The Cocaine-Snorting Organ Donor

Organ transplants are some of the most amazing surgeries. I've always wondered how they can attach every part of an organ into a new body and actually make it work. The answer may be simpler than you think. For example, the kidney basically has three tubes attached to it. One is an artery that supplies blood from the heart to the kidney. The second is a vein that takes the blood out of the kidney and back to the heart. As blood passes through the kidney, waste products are filtered out to create urine, which comes out of the third tube, called the ureter, which is attached to the bladder. And there you have it, the body's very own purification system. All you have to do during a transplant is attach the artery of the new kidney to an artery in the body, the vein to a vein, and stick the ureter into the patient's bladder, and you're done. The process of putting a kidney into a new body takes all of 45 minutes in the hands of an experienced surgeon. It's pretty amazing.

An exciting part of the transplant surgery rotation is that the surgery team sometimes goes to other hospitals to operate on the donating body in order to obtain the organs. It's called a procurement, and if a student is lucky, they'll get to fly on a private jet to some far off destination to pick up an organ. On my final day of the transplant surgery rotation, we had a procurement. Unfortunately, it was only 20 minutes down the road at a local hospital, so no private jet was necessary. Nonetheless, I was looking forward to seeing what happens on the donation side of transplant surgery. By the time we got the call, the donor's blood type was already matched, and the potential recipients already identified. The soon-to-be recipients of these organs had received the long awaited phone call at 5AM…"Your kidney is on the way, come to the hospital immediately for surgery." The process of matching donors to recipients is a complicated one. It involves ranking potential recipients on a list based on their current health, then waiting for the right donor to come along that matches them well enough to actually serve as a donor.

The process could take years. So, as you can imagine, it's a special day when people find out they are finally getting their organ. So these patients started on their way that morning, some from four or more hours away, to get to the hospital for the operation, not having much time to think or prepare. And as these patients began their journey towards the hospital for long awaited organs, we began our road trip to the nearby hospital. The deceased donor turned out to be a drug addict who had overdosed on cocaine the night before and was now brain dead after having a large stroke. He had been kept on a breathing machine in order to make sure his organs were getting enough oxygen to keep them alive and functioning. His heart was still pumping blood. But the patient was very much dead.

The process of cutting out the donor's organs began with a long incision all the way down his chest and abdomen. Our team was in charge of the abdominal organs (kidneys, liver, and pancreas), and another team would come in later for the heart and lungs. This order made sense, because taking out the heart and lungs first would leave the other organs without circulating blood and oxygen which could cause unnecessary damage. The process was slow...very slow. Each artery and vein had to be cut and tied off just right to ensure it could be placed properly into the new body. Four hours into the surgery, and we had yet to take out a single organ. It was just a lot of dissecting and clipping. At around the fifth hour, the heart/lung surgeon came in to check on our progress. But as he spoke with us, he noticed a small area on the lungs that looked funny, and asked us to take a quick biopsy (or piece of tissue) from the lung to have it looked at by a pathologist under a microscope. The tissue was sent away, and within 10 minutes, the pathologist came into the room and made the disappointing announcement.

"It's a small cell."

What that meant was this patient actually had cancer, a type of cancer known as small cell carcinoma. It doesn't sound good, and it isn't. This meant that we could not use any of the organs, because this cancer may have already spread to them. It would be truly unfortunate to accidentally give cancer to an organ recipient. Unfortunately, this meant we had just wasted four hours on a Saturday morning cutting open a human body for no reason at all. But this was nothing compared to what had to happen next.

Back at our hospital, two families were anxiously waiting. They had been called early that morning and told that today, they would get their long-awaited kidney. We walked into the private waiting room, and with a somber and compassionate look, the surgeon broke the bad news.

"Unfortunately, it turns out that the donor had cancer that no one knew about, so you won't be getting that kidney today. So, go home, stay healthy, and chances are your name will come up again soon."

A part of me was expecting these people to blow up..."HOW COULD YOU NOT KNOW THIS! I DROVE 4 HOURS AT 5AM THIS MORNING!!!" But the response was quite different. It was almost a sense of relief. I didn't understand it at first, but it began making sense later. These people had suffered for years with their kidney failure, going for dialysis every other day, and at some point, it must have become a way of life. Sure a kidney would be great, but it would also mean a huge surgery. And that's not all. Just because you get a kidney doesn't mean you are cured. In fact, you are merely switching one disease for another, because after you get the new organ, you now have to take tons of drugs to weaken your immune system so that your body doesn't reject the new organ. So, for the rest of their lives, organ recipients are "immuno-compromised". Not an easy way to live, since you are much more likely to get sick. There was undoubtedly some disappointment mixed in with their relief, but in the end, I don't think they minded waiting a bit longer.

Despite this difficult day, my transplant surgery experience overall was amazing. It was my first real appreciation of how far medicine has come, and the amazing things we are capable of doing. But it also taught me that medicine has its limitations. There is only so much we can do for those that suffer from afflictions like kidney failure, and unfortunately, there really is no "cure", not even transplant. But as the years go by, more of these limitations will turn into opportunities to advance medicine. Who knows what is in store down the road – artificial kidneys made by the thousands in factories, a robotic arm for an amputee that actually moves when the patient thinks about moving it, small armies of molecule-sized drugs that go through your body and destroy only cancerous cells. It may surprise you that some of this is already in the works. It truly is an amazing time to be in medicine.

Chapter 8

Saying Goodbye

Ask the typical medical student why they went into medicine, and the answer is usually the same. It's some variation of, "I want to help people." What is often hard for us to realize early in our careers is that while we may be able to help many people and watch them walk out of the hospital, there are many others that aren't as lucky. I learned this lesson very quickly one night during an eight hour emergency room shift.

I was scheduled to be in the ER for the night shift, which was from midnight to 8AM. It was usually a pretty good shift to work, as business tended to be the slowest at night. During my previous night shifts, I spent most of my time reading email. But this particular night would prove to be different. The first bit of excitement was an infant that arrived in cardiac arrest. The story was that the infant was found not breathing by her mother, and the ambulance crew had already performed CPR for 45 minutes before their arrival to the hospital without much luck. I kept my distance when the infant arrived, as over 15 medical team members, including pediatric residents, the emergency room attendings, and critical care nurses, all squeezed in to surround this tiny body. It appeared that this was a case of SIDS (sudden infant death syndrome) and the infant's chances of survival were slim at best. But the team worked relentlessly, putting in IVs, performing chest compressions and administering drugs to get her little heart pumping again. Then, ten minutes into the resuscitation, two people with the most devastated looks on their faces came walking into the room – the child's parents. The mother was frantic, and was yelling, "Please save my baby!" The father held his wife, and cried quietly. I had no idea parents or family members were allowed into the room during these resuscitations. The staff gave them a chair, and they were allowed to sit and watch as the medical team worked frantically. But despite the team's efforts, the baby died. I can't imagine what must have been going through the parents' minds, and at the time truly wondered if having them in the room was good for either the parents or for the medical team trying to save the child.

Later in the course of the night came multiple trauma patients. One came in by helicopter from another hospital, and with him came some x-rays. He had been in a terrible car accident. I had the job of running the x-rays to the radiologist to find out what bones were broken while the rest of the team dealt with the patient. He had so many broken bones, I had to write them all down so I wouldn't forget any when I relayed the message to the team. He survived long enough to make it out of the ER and into the intensive care unit.

The patients just kept on coming that night. As a medical student, we have the privilege of being able to walk into virtually any interesting case, and have the luxury of not really being responsible for anything, because everyone assumes that we know nothing. So, off I went into another interesting case. It was an 81 year old man who was found unconscious by his family. But as EMS rolled him into the room, he was sitting up and attempting to communicate. Unfortunately, he only spoke Greek, so we were unsure of what he was saying. He looked extremely frightened, and in the middle of his sentence, stopped speaking, and slumped over unconscious. The team immediately began the resuscitation. His clothes were stripped off, IVs were placed, and medications were given. EKG leads were stuck onto his chest, and a needle was placed through his chest and next to his heart in an attempt to drain fluid that was thought to be building up. A tube was placed down his throat to help him breath. Two lines were placed in his femoral arteries very close to his groin. Chest compressions were started, and after a few minutes, the emergency room physician looked over at me, and calmly said, "You ready?" He wanted me to do chest compressions! I was, in fact, ready. Finally, a chance to actually help out. So, I stepped onto a small stool next to the stretcher, leaned over the body, and began pressing my body weight into this frail man's chest, fearing I would soon feel ribs popping under my hands. Mercifully, I did not. This continued for at least ten minutes before I heard the dreaded words... "The family is here, they would like to come in." Here I was, beating on an old man, a naked man that had tubes coming out of everywhere, and they were going to let the family see this?! And indeed, there they were, the wife, and the son. The wife was obviously distressed, and she immediately walked to the head of the bed amidst the chaos and sat beside him, crying, stroking his face, talking to him in Greek. She seemed to be oblivious to the lines and tubes, she saw only him. I looked at the attending, hoping to get the sign to stop, and he did indeed tell me it was okay to stop. He turned to the wife and put his hand on her small shoulder.

"I'm sorry, we've lost him."

We eventually left the room, and allowed her to be alone with her husband.

In the course of 8 hours that night, four of our patients had died. It was more death than I had ever thought I would see. I dealt with it better than expected, not letting it truly bother me until my drive home, when I began thinking of all the people that had lost their loved ones that night. A mother had lost her child. A wife had lost her husband of over 50 years. That's when it hurt. I sat and thought about how the families had the chance to be with their loved ones during their final minutes of life. Although I had my doubts at first, the elderly couple convinced me that this was the right thing to do. She got a chance to be with her husband and say her final goodbye during his last moments. And although our fancy cardiac monitors would have us believe he had probably passed away before she even came into the room, something in me believes he heard her say goodbye.

In the end, it seems like what people need most is some sort of closure. Although terrifying, letting family bear witness allows them to realize that everything possible was done for their loved one. But more importantly, it gives them a chance to say goodbye. I can't imagine denying anyone that chance.

Chapter 9

The Reoccurring Refrigerator Incident

Exposing students to actual patients is something most medical schools try to do as early as possible. These early encounters allow students to develop a sense of comfort in what can often be an unsettling environment. After all, we as students are probing into the health problems of patients, as well as examining their bodies, two very personal matters for a patient. So, it makes sense to get students out there early, and allow them to get adjusted to this new environment.

During the first semester of medical school, we spent a small amount of time each week in a course designed to teach us the intangibles of the patient-doctor interaction…how to talk with patients, how to give bad news, and how to be compassionate caregivers. They even hired local actors who played the role of fake patients and allowed us to interview them for practice. When the second half of our first year came around, we were finally allowed to see the doctor-patient relationship in action by shadowing a physician in clinic. I was paired with a family medicine doctor. Looking back, it's obvious that my view of medicine at the time was the "bright-eyed and bushy-tailed" version where doctors were always compassionate and caring, and addressed each patient's problems with enthusiasm. As the day started, it was living up to this, as the doctor saw only a few patients and was able to spend the time to address even their minor issues. As we got midway through the afternoon, we stepped out of a patient room, only to be confronted by a frantic nurse. The patient in the next room was seizing. The doctor, unphased, slowly made his way to the room. We entered together, and sure enough, there was a woman in the corner, sitting in her chair, making jerking movements of all her extremities, appearing to be unresponsive, while her sister stood beside her, trying to comfort her. The doctor looked at them for about one second, then went and calmly sat in the opposite corner and started looking over her file. I was in disbelief. "Shouldn't you do something?" I thought to myself. Why didn't he care? This woman was in obvious distress. Eventually, the seizure stopped, and her sister sat down and began discussing how these episodes happen multiple times each day. The doctor, still busy reading the file, didn't even look up, so the woman directed most of her comments at me. I was obviously concerned for them and listened attentively and she picked up on this. Finally, the doctor began talking, cutting her off mid-sentence…

"So what do you want?"

There was no compassion in his voice, but a cold, matter-of-factness that made me uncomfortable to be in the room.

"Well, we're out of her pain medication, and she needs more. She's in so much pain."

"Did you go to the pain clinic like I asked you to?"

Again, the doctor's voice was cutting, and now bordering on accusatory. I couldn't believe what I was hearing. This woman was obviously suffering, her sister was trying to help, and here was a doctor who apparently didn't care.

"No, we never had a chance, but we're planning on going there next week."

The woman seemed very genuine, and her sister was looking much better following her seizure, and began participating in the conversation as well.

"Yes, I'm definitely going to go as soon as I can find some time. But I just need some medication until I can get there."

With this, the doctor abruptly got up, and headed for the door.

"Let me see what I can do."

We both left the room and went back to his office. I wanted to stand up for this patient. I wanted to yell at the doctor, "Why are you treating them like this?! This patient needs you!" Where was the compassion I had heard so much about? But before I had a chance to question what I had just seen, the doctor said the two words that would slap the bright-eyed picture of medicine out of my system forever...

"She's faking."

Just having started medical school, I did not yet have the knowledge to appreciate a medical con artist at work. But anyone with medical training would have seen this patient and realized that all was not as it seemed. For example, true full-blown seizures, such as this woman was apparently having, are followed by long periods of excessive fatigue or sleep, and the patients never return to normal right after the event. Second, generalized seizures lead to loss of consciousness, making it nearly impossible for them to actually stay seated in a chair during the event.

And lastly, and perhaps most importantly, pain medication is not a treatment for seizures, so asking for pain medication to prevent a patient's convulsions screams, "I'm a drug addict" to any doctor.

"They come here all the time," the physician continued, "always asking for pain medications. They're both abusing it. The sister has a known history of drug abuse. Those aren't seizures you saw. It's all an act."

The very next year, while spending a month working on the inpatient neurology service, the attending asked that I go evaluate a new patient whom they suspected had pseudoseizures. This phenomenon occurs when a patient appears to be having a seizure, but when hooked up to electrodes on their heads, the firing of neurons that are present with real seizures is not present. These events are usually triggered by stressful situations, and often come along with a history of prior abuse. No one is quite sure whether patients intentionally have pseudoseizures. Most believe that even though they aren't a result of true organic pathology, in a way, it is still out of the patient's control. It is the body's unconscious way of dealing with a stressor, similar to having a headache when we are stressed. This particular patient had recently revealed to his family that he was gay, and it had not gone over well. While at work, he had an apparent seizure. So,

51

I went in to examine the patient, and as we were talking, he went into a spell, with arms thrashing all over the place and hips thrusting off the bed. By this point I had seen true seizures, and I knew this wasn't it. He was already hooked up to electrodes to determine if he really was having seizures, and to no surprise, there was no increase in firing from his brain, leading to the diagnosis of pseudoseizures. He was discharged that afternoon, with an appointment to see a psychiatrist.

By the time I was a fourth year, I had all but forgotten these two incidents, and once again began taking things at face value. That was until I started my emergency medicine rotation.

The emergency department is an interesting place. There are those that come in with real problems, such as chest pain and lacerations in need of stitches. But the vast majority fit under the non-acute category. These are the people that come in with issues that belong in their regular doctor's office, such as rashes, ear aches, diarrhea, and even trouble sleeping. These are not emergencies. And finally, there are those people that do not belong in any medical facility. These are the most frustrating to deal with.

It was getting late in the evening when a new patient's name popped up on our computer system indicating he needed to be evaluated. Under the reason for visit, it read, "back injury". I found him outside in the hallway (all of the other rooms were full), waiting on a stretcher. He was in obvious discomfort. He could barely lift his hand to shake mine as I introduced myself.

"What brings you in here today?"

He winced as he replied, "I've hurt my back. I was helping my son lift a refrigerator and heard a pop in my back, and it's been killing me ever since."

I asked him the various questions that might indicate he herniated a disc.

"Do you feel pain down your leg?"

"Yeh, it feels like lightning shooting all the way down. I can barely move."

"Any trouble using the bathroom or numbness in your thighs?"

"No, just can't move, I'm in so much pain."

I examined him, lifting each leg and watching him as he writhed around in pain.

"Have you ever hurt your back like this before?"

"No, I've had some back pain from a car accident, but this is different. Never hurt it like this."

And then came the line that every ER physician hates to hear:

"I think I'm going to need some vicodin. I'm allergic to almost everything else. It's the only thing that works for my pain."

This man had all the signs of a drug seeker. He knew the name of what he wanted, he knew exactly how to describe his back pain without prompting us to do further testing like an MRI, he was "allergic" to everything else, and he had a good story. Being somewhat naïve, I bought his story, and went back to the attending doctor to tell him of my findings, convinced this man needed some strong pain medications. I began telling my story to the doctor, but before I could finish, he had pulled up an ER report from the same patient a year earlier. The report read, "Patient presents with back pain after lifting his refrigerator earlier today..." I had been duped.

Patients who are addicted to pain medicine end up going from doctor to doctor with their story in hopes of scoring narcotics. Once the doctor is on to them and stops prescribing medicine or tries referring them to pain clinics for further help, the patient disappears, and ends up at another doctor's office. It's a very sad thing. This patient was undoubtedly going from ER to ER with his story, hoping someone would buy it. He probably forgot he had already used the story at our ER, or maybe he didn't know we kept electronic records.

As we walked back together to see the patient, the competitor in me was hoping the attending would tell him he had lost in his attempt to trick us, and that he should not go to ERs because it was a huge waste of taxpayer money and everyone's time. But he simply went up to him, said we could give him one dose of medicine since he was in the ER, but that he needed to go to his regular doctor for a prescription. He was an experienced ER doctor, one could even say he was a bit jaded, because he knew there was no need to waste his breath or any more of his time. No matter what he said, this man would just simply go somewhere else and try again. Such is the way of addiction. So, no, we did not win this battle. In fact, we were all losers, in one way or another.

The patient figured his scheme was not working, and did not make any argument. The nurse brought him his medicine, and I went back to let him know he was free to go. As I left him to go see my next patient, I looked back in time to catch a glimpse of him walking comfortably out the door.

I learned a great deal from these three patients. First, I learned to be a bit more critical of patients, a lesson I wish I had not learned. Second, I learned that problems you can't simply fix with medicines are harder to treat, and often more disabling for patients. Finally, I learned that there comes a time in every medical student's life when they realize medicine is not quite what they had imagined. For me, no longer was medicine always about the grateful patient, the dedicated doctor, and the disease we would fight together.

Chapter 10
Mistakes

People expect a lot from their doctors. They expect honesty and openness, they expect treatment, and they expect results. One thing no one expects is a mistake. After all, doctors don't make mistakes, right? Well, like any other human being, doctors make lots of mistakes. Even the best doctors make mistakes. Allow me to demonstrate.

I take you once again to my ophthalmology rotation. For an entire week, my assignment was to work with one of the most well-known ophthalmologist in the state, and quite possibly, the country. Patients took trips from all over the nation just to see him for a 20 minute clinic visit. In the medicine world, he was a rock star. For an entire week, I saw him handle some of the most complex cases with confidence and ease. In the OR, he was like a machine, going through case after case of small, delicate eye surgery. Then one day, I learned he too was human. An African-American woman was having surgery on her eye muscles to correct her "lazy eye". They initially sedated her, and then performed what is known as retrobulbar anesthesia. For this, a needle is inserted through the eyelid and behind the eye, where the anesthesia liquid is injected. This inactivates all of the nerves that run behind your eye, both the sensory nerves and the motor nerves. Since your sensory nerves are no longer functioning, you don't feel any pain. You also can no longer see anything, since vision travels along special sensory nerves. The motor nerves control eye movement, so you can't move your eyes either. In essence, that eye is useless for about eight hours after the injection.

In the OR, to ensure that the proper eye is operated on, the person's face would have a big "X" drawn with a marker on the forehead over the correct eye. But on this day, the "X" had been partially obscured by the sterile drapes that covered the patient for the operation. The ophthalmologist grabbed the needle with the anesthesia, and carefully inserted it in her left eye. It was only after he finished that the anesthesiologist pointed to the "X" on the right side of her forehead. Everyone stopped, and the ophthalmologist stood there in disbelief. The small amount of his face that was visible behind the mask and surgical cap was turning redder by the second. He walked over to the patient's chart, still in disbelief. But it was true, he had completely anesthetized the wrong eye.

I expected him to say something humble, taking responsibility for the mistake. Instead, he started mumbling about how the anesthesiologist usually sits on the side opposite the eye to be operated on, and how the anesthesiologist was on the wrong side, and that's why he made the mistake. "Bullshit," I thought to myself.

Was it truly a big deal? After all, he hadn't started operating yet. That would have truly been tragic. But now, the other eye for this patient would have to be numbed up, and that would mean the patient would be totally blind for the rest of the day! That could be a problem. They needed permission to do this to the patient, and so the doctor left the OR in hopes that her mother or father were in the waiting room. Unfortunately, only an uncle had come with her, and he wasn't allowed to give permission for this. So, the patient had to be woken up out of sedation and told of the mistake. She could then decide to come back another day, or agree to inject the other eye and be temporarily blind. So, the anesthesiologist started reversing the sedation, and we waited for her to become fully alert. When she was finally awake, the doctor broke the news to her.

"It appears we made a mistake, and you got the numbing medicine in the wrong eye."

She responded with a very appropriate question, "Isn't there a big 'X' over my right eye?"

Yup, there sure was, and the doctor had still injected the wrong eye. In the end, she agreed to proceed with the operation, even though it meant she'd need a close assistant all day to guide her around.

Unfortunately, the patient wasn't the only blind one in the operating room that day. Mistakes happen. Everyone makes them. But you've got to see that you've made a mistake and learn from it, or else you're likely to make the same one again.

Chapter 11

Big Pimping

Mention the word to anybody in medicine, and they'll know exactly what it means. No, it has nothing to do with a cane, a sparkling sports coat, and the exploitation of women. The world of medicine has a completely different definition of pimping. It's the process in which those that are higher in the medicine hierarchy ask their subordinates questions on various topics in medicine to test their knowledge. Most of the pimping is directed towards medical students. There are three main reasons that an attending or senior resident would pimp medical students. And here they are...

Reason 1: The True Teacher

The first reason is probably the best reason to pimp. Many attendings ask very reasonable questions simply to see what a student's level of knowledge is, and if the student does not know the answer to a particular question, the attending uses this to delve into a brief teaching session. The truly attentive physician will preface his/her question with an "outie". This "outie" is a phrase that prevents you from feeling stupid in case you don't know the answer. Examples of outies include, "I really don't expect you to know this, but..." or, "One thousand bonus points if you can tell me..." This is a great way of pimping.

Reason 2: The Showoff

I'm convinced that some physicians like to pimp just so they have a reason to show off their medical knowledge. They'll ask very specific questions, such as, "What are the diagnostic criteria for endocarditis?" The question is usually very matter-of-fact, as if everyone should know the answer, and he simply wants you to share, since you of course know it as well. And when you don't know the answer, the physician fakes a small bit of surprise, and then goes into a long-winded discussion on the topic, including the recent data on the subject. Not a fun way of pimping students, as they are usually too embarrassed that they didn't know the answer to truly pay attention to the teaching session that follows.

Reason 3: Searching for the next Ms. Cleo

The worst of all the pimpers are the ones who ask the unanswerable questions. No matter how much you know, there is no way to answer their questions. Attendings are, in essence, asking you to read their minds. These are the questions like, "Tell me what four things you worry about in this patient," when it is a patient who happens to have 20 medical problems. Sometimes, the question is often prefaced with, "This is a read-my-mind kind of question, but…". If those words come out of your mouth, don't ask the question! Don't do it. It's just silly. I've told myself that when I become an attending, my questions will all be for the sole purpose of teaching students in a comfortable environment. Although, just for fun, I will stand around one morning, with my bright-eyed and bushy-tailed students, who are expecting all this knowledge and intellectual questioning to come out of my mouth. Instead, I'll just point to the one that looks the most nervous and say, "You! What am I thinking right now?"

Chapter 12

Reading Between the Lines

P=MD. It was an equation passed down to us by classes that came before. This simply meant that since our medical school was graded on an honors/pass/fail grading system, all we had to do was pass everything to earn our MD degree. And since it was surprisingly difficult to fail courses so long as you gave some effort, this made it seem like medical school would be a cakewalk. But in reality, things were not as simple as P=MD. Almost every member of our class wanted to pursue a specialty, and finding a residency spot can be quite the competitive process, so grades did matter.

Getting good grades in high school and college was never a problem for those in my class. They would not have made it into medical school without being able to perform on tests. Our basic science courses during our first year were like our college courses on speed. We covered insane amounts of material in short periods of time. But at the end of the day, it was still the same old, same old. Your grades were based on how easily you could memorize material and how compulsively you wanted to study.

But as we got closer to the real world, the way we were graded began to change. After our first year in the classroom, we entered the hospital and began working on the ward teams. The majority of your grade was based on the subjective evaluation by residents and attendings. Suddenly, scales such as "professionalism" and "ability to work with peers" determined your grade, something new to everyone. It was those that were socially adept that now found themselves a step ahead of the bookworms.

In such an environment, you always have to be careful of what you say. It becomes very important to come across as enthusiastic and interested in learning. This can sometimes be difficult, given the situation. Here are two examples:

Situation 1 – It's time to go home. The typical medical student will stay in the hospital until the upper level resident tells them they should leave. Sometimes, the residents get so busy that they lose track of the time, and forget that the students are still around. But when it's 6PM and you've done a whole lot of nothing all day, and you're ready to go home, it's a tough balance between hinting that you want to go home, and not sounding like you want to go home. After all, the perfect medical student would never want to leave early. Some of my classmates would just suck it up and wait around until getting permission to go home. The minority would leave without checking in with the resident. For me, it came down to expressing my enthusiasm, yet subtly reminding the resident that I was still around and had nothing to do. During my first year on the wards, I would usually say something like, "What else can I help you with?" It was an easy way to express enthusiasm while reminding the resident I had nothing to do. Worked every time.

Situation 2 – Scut work. Scut work is the kind of work that has to be done around the hospital that a well-trained monkey could do. Most residents are good about not giving medical students this type of work, since it's bad form on their part. After all, students are paying to be there, and we're supposed to be learning, not doing crap work. But sometimes, there is just too much going on, and there is nothing else for the students to do. So we bravely rise to the challenge of scut. But when we are asked to help with scut work, it is again important to come across as enthusiastic about the task, so as not to show our lack of interest. So, when the resident asks, "Hey (insert med student name here), could you run these x-rays down to the file room for me?", the correct response is, "I'd be more than happy too." Or, "Hey student, can you call this patient's pharmacy and get his medication list?" "Sure, I'd love to do that." Sometimes, the task calls for a slightly modified response. The resident may ask, "Hey student, can you go do a rectal exam on Mr. Jones in Room 12?" In this situation, the typical, "I'd be more than happy too" sounds a little creepy. The more moderate, "No problem, I'll take care of it" usually suffices.

This all sounds a little silly, I know. After all, does it really matter exactly how you ask to leave, or respond to scut work? Well, in retrospect, it probably doesn't matter much at all, so long as the resident knows you're working hard. But as a student, you feel like you are constantly under the spotlight, and every move is being watched and noted. Even small things, like having a resident see you checking email during the day can make you feel as if you just lost a few points. For many students, this constant obsession with looking dedicated and seeking good evaluations is almost a pathologic disease. It is a very real phenomenon, and it seems to affect students across the board, although they often display the signs and symptoms differently. It's almost a constant discomfort in one's own skin. They promptly stand up to offer their seats to residents, they feel the constant compulsion to take notes when attendings are talking, and they nod in agreement with every comment. They apologize profusely if even a little late, they present patients for much too long and give too many details. It is this constant unease that distinguishes the medical students in every environment.

Maybe we hold ourselves to an unreasonable standard, which inevitably makes life that much harder on the wards. I eventually learned to relax, and just act like my normal self. It was this normal self that got along well with others. This normal self was the social achiever, and my grades reflected my ability to get along more than they did my academic prowess.

By the fourth year, students transform into more comfortable creatures, and our whole language changes. We no longer make residents read between the lines. The question changes from, "Is there anything else I can do," to, "I'm gonna take off, unless there is something you need." This change comes with time, and every medical student goes through some level of attitude change while on the wards. It's exhausting to keep your guard up for two whole years. Eventually, you learn to relax a little, truly enjoy your time on the wards, and let the grades simply come as they may.

Chapter 13

Blood and Gore

I walked into the operating room, and found my way into a corner. For this surgery, I was to be only an observer. The operation was underway, and the patient's abdomen had already been cut open. There was a small curtain that separated the lower half of the body from the upper, so I couldn't see the patient's face. There were large retractors that were hooked under the skin and pulled back, allowing for a better view of the inside of the body. The surgeon continued cutting, skillfully using a bovie (an object that looks like a pen that sends current through the tip, thereby burning shut the bleeding vessels it touches). The surgeons were all wearing full body protection, from the facemask all the way down to shoe covers. They were expecting this one to be messy.

A small incision was made deeper into the abdomen, which I couldn't see. Fluid came gushing out, and spilled over the side of the body, along with blood and various particles of tissue. Had they made a mistake and hit the bladder or stomach? I couldn't believe this patient was still alive. It seemed like she had already lost so much blood, and now something appeared to have exploded inside her. Just when I thought it couldn't get any worse, two of the surgeons grabbed hold of something deep in the belly, and began pulling in opposite directions. They put their entire weight into it, leaning back while holding onto some part of the woman's body. The tissue gave way, and the horrendous sounds of human tissue tearing could be heard above the din of the anesthesia machines. Surely this was the end for this patient. It seemed like they were killing her!

"Doing okay?" the doctor asked.

"I'm fine," came a small voice from behind the curtain.

"Oh my god," I thought to myself. "This patient is actually awake!"

The attending gave the nearby intern a nod, and the intern immediately fell forward onto the lower chest of the patient, bearing down with all her weight. This was no small intern either. This would surely be the final blow. And, as the intern bore down on this poor woman who continued to bleed profusely, the attending surgeon dug his entire hand into the open abdomen, felt around, and pulled out what appeared to be an alien life form covered in creamy goo and blood. The creature let out a piercing scream, announcing his arrival. The baby had been born.

I had no idea that a caesarian section would be so gruesome. I still can't believe the human body can live through something that appears so traumatic. After making the initial small incision, the surgeons literally tear open the uterus. Amniotic fluid rushes out, which is the swimming pool that the fetus has called home for nine months. The pressure applied to the upper abdomen helps pop the fetus out of the uterus. All the while, the patient is usually awake throughout the procedure! Thanks to anesthesia, she feels no pain. They do hold up a drape to separate the patient's head from the abdomen, so the mother (and father that may be present) cannot see the war zone. Good thing. The experience left me feeling truly fortunate to be a male, although I developed an undying respect for women and all they go through in life, including the miracle of childbirth.

Chapter 14
The Explosion

During our first year on the wards, we go through what is known as the "core" rotations. These allow us to work in the various fields of medicine that are the basics of general care. The core rotations at most schools include surgery, internal medicine, pediatrics, obstetrics/gynecology, psychiatry, family medicine, and neurology. Each rotation typically lasts between one and two months. During our surgery rotation, we spent two days in the ER, working alongside the surgery resident who was called whenever an ER case came in that could require surgical intervention. These were always the most interesting cases in the ER. The first case I saw was a hunter who had been shot by a rifle from very close range. His side had been towards the gunman, and the bullet went into his upper back, tunneled under the skin of his back, and left a large exit crater behind his shoulder. By the time we got to him, he was loaded up with morphine, and requesting a Snickers® bar. Amazing stuff, that morphine. The surgery resident proceeded to shove gauze dressing down into the tunnel the bullet had left. This served to put some pressure on the bleeding areas to prevent him from losing too much blood. Lucky for this guy, the bullet completely missed his spinal cord and most of the vital structures in his body. It had mostly just torn through the fat on his back, of which he had a pretty good supply. He was very lucky that night.

The second case was one I will never forget, or at least my nose will never forget. I was asked to go see this patient on my own initially, then discuss him with the resident. Entering the room, I saw a couple that was probably in their mid 50's. The husband was laying on the table, not appearing to be in any distress.

"What brings you in today, sir."

"I have this large mass on my belly, and it's been getting larger for a few weeks now. I figured it was time to get it looked at."

If there is one thing I've learned, it's that some people wait inordinately large amounts of time with seemingly awful states of health, knowing full well that something is wrong, but just assuming that if they wait long enough, it'll go away. Well, the mass on his stomach was now the size of a grapefruit, and it had become quite obvious that it wasn't going away. To make matters worse, the mass was exquisitely painful, severely limiting his activity.

I continued to get his story, including his past medical history. Apparently, he had a small area like this come up in the same place many years ago, but it seemed to go away on its own (which probably helped him take the "watch and wait" approach). After getting the story, it was time to take a look at his belly. Sure enough, there was this large, elevated mass on his right lower abdomen, with an area in the middle that looked as if it had a very thin layer of skin, with blood pooling underneath. I pressed on the mass gently, and in the middle, there was an area that felt...well... squishy, which was an indication that he likely had a big pool of pus sitting underneath. I left the room, and told the resident the story.

"It's probably an abscess," he told me. "We will have to open it up."

The resident was still busy tending to the gunshot victim, so I went back to the room to share our plan with the patient. As I entered, there was an unusual smell that was initially faint, but began getting stronger as the seconds went by. It smelled like rotten eggs.

"Do you smell that," I asked.

The man took a deep breath. "Yeh, what is that?" I looked down at the man's stomach and noticed that his gown had become slightly wet in the area of his right lower abdomen. I put on gloves, and carefully lifted his gown. Sure enough, the ball of pus finally could not hold itself, and had started to ooze out from the center.

"Oh my!" His wife looked a little scared.

"Well, looks like it popped. We're going to have to give it a good squeeze to get this pus out," I told him.

All this while, the smell kept getting stronger and stronger. It was the worst thing I had smelled in my entire life. In fact, the smell was leaking out of the room and into the rest of the ER.

I stepped out to get some more gauze, ready to get as much pus out of this thing as possible. The nurses outside had begun noticing the odor, and asked me what was going on.

"His big ball of pus just exploded." His nurse walked into his room, and a few seconds later, had to walk out. The smell was just too much. She had to leave the ER and walk outside for a while, sure she was about to vomit. ER nurses have seen it all, and if they can't handle a smell, you better believe it's bad.

I tried to be brave and walked back in. The only way to do this was to breathe through my mouth, in hopes of avoiding the unpleasantness. I went to work, pressing firmly on the sides of the mass, as the pus and blood began pouring through the top. With each push, the patient grimaced in obvious pain, and more yellow liquid came seeping out. I wiped it as quickly as I could with the gauze, and soon realized I was running out and would need to go get even more. Good thing, as the stench was beginning to seep into my nose regardless of how hard I tried to breathe through my mouth. It was again becoming unbearable. My words came out extra breathy, trying hard not to let any air flow through the nostrils.

"Ahh'll be bhack in just a sec."

I got outside, and it was obvious that the smell had now seeped into half of the ER, as everyone was standing around, holding their noses, wondering what was happening. There were a few patients that were in the hallways (which is where they're kept if all the rooms are full). The poor woman who was assigned the spot outside of this particular room was losing it as well. The only saving grace was a small bottle of wintergreen scented liquid that the nurses were passing around. This was super-concentrated stuff, which I assume was used by putting a few drops into bad smelling stuff. This poor patient squeezed multiple drops onto her fingers and then proceeded to smear it right onto her upper lip.

Overuse of this scented liquid had left the area smelling of wintergreen pus. It was horrendous. The nurse that had to walk out earlier came back and told me how I was her hero for actually going into the war zone. Another medical student that was working with me walked up, and offered to help. I let him go back in there to squeeze the rest of the juice out of the grapefruit. The smell had become unbearable for me, and I couldn't go back in.

Turns out, the man had his appendix removed when he was younger, and the stitches they used to sew up his skin had been metal ones that never dissolved. Any foreign object in the body is bad news, as it can serve as a place for bacteria to hold on to and set up camp, allowing them to multiply within the body. Unfortunately for this man, the surgeons decided that they would not be able to remove all the stitches for reasons that are still unclear to me. Although they were able to fully drain his abscess, it would likely happen to him again at some point. I'm assuming he won't wait as long to seek help next time.

As for me and the other student that helped drain the abscess, we could smell the odor on our white coats that entire night. As soon as I arrived home, I threw everything in the washer, and as I was about to enter the shower, I could still distinctly smell the abscess. Maybe it was just in my head I thought, but then raised my arm and took a good whiff of my forearm. The scent had actually gotten into my skin!!! I must have scrubbed myself down for an hour. For months after this incident, I would see my fellow medical student every now and then, and our conversation would consist of the same two lines:

"Man, that thing was nasty."

"Dude, so nasty."

There is little delay in seeking medical attention when your problem is as dramatic as a gunshot wound. But there are problems just as life-threatening that come on so slowly, we are able to keep convincing ourselves that everything is okay. Lives would be saved for cancer patients and infections could be treated before they rage out of control, simply by getting help sooner rather than later. Therefore, I have developed a simple system to determine when it is time to seek medical help. Just ask yourself, "If I went up to a complete stranger and told them about my medical problem, would they think everything is alright?" If the answer is "no", go see a doctor. I guarantee a stranger will never give you an "all-clear" when you've got a grapefruit-sized ball of pus in your belly.

Chapter 15

The Medical Student

A young couple sits outside of a corner coffee shop. It's early, and cars busily hustle by, carrying people to their places of work. About half an hour into their morning coffee, the observant woman sees a familiar car pass by. "I think that's the third time that guy has passed this corner," she says to her husband. The husband barely looks over his morning newspaper, and with a casual glance, is back into the sports section. "Maybe he's lost," he replies, settling further into his chair.

But for the man in this car, his morning is not so relaxing. And no, it's not his third time driving by the same corner, it's his twelfth. He is not lost. On the contrary, he knows these roads better than perhaps anyone in his town. He is late for work once again, but continues circling around the block. The reason is simple -- he can't stop.

This is a typical morning for our troubled driver. Every morning he comes down this road. Right before reaching the coffee shop, he runs over a patch of uneven road. He knows it's coming, he passes it every day. But no matter how hard he tries, the minute his car runs over this patch of road, the same thought comes barreling through, knocking away anything else in his mind.

"Did I just run somebody over?"

The rational mind says it's very unlikely. After all, he looked in his rearview mirror and saw no one laying in the road, just the familiar uneven pavement. He runs over the same pavement each day, and today was no different. There is no look of panic on the pedestrians walking by as if an accident just happened. But another voice in his head thunders over rationality, and convinces him that anything is possible. So, around the block he circles, and passes the same road again. His anxiety is relieved when he sees no one laying in the street, no terrified pedestrians calling 911 frantically. But he again drives over the same rough patch, and again thoughts of ambulances and an injured man are back, so he circles again, just to be sure.

This is the mind of someone who suffers from obsessive-compulsive disorder (OCD), one of the most fascinating and devastating conditions in psychiatry. I saw a number of patients with this disease during my psychiatry rotation. There are two distinct parts to this disorder. The first is the obsession, which is an irrational, intruding thought. For our driver, it's the thought that he may have run someone over. For others, it can be worries about germs, constant fear that the stove was left on, or an irrational belief that something bad will happen if their sock drawer is disheveled. Interestingly, these people often realize their thoughts are irrational, but these thoughts continue to dominate their day. This obsession is followed by a compulsion, which is a physical action that relieves the stress brought about by the obsession. In our examples, that would be constantly circling the block, washing your hands 100 times a day, constantly checking and rechecking the stove, or making sure your socks are perfectly arranged. However, in order for these thoughts and actions to be considered a disorder, it has to adversely affect the person's ability to function. Whether it be trouble at work, difficulty in personal relationships, or trouble with the law, it has to negatively impact one's life. Unfortunately, these people are labeled as "crazy" for their affliction. They are treated by psychiatrists and medications.

There is a very similar type of person in society, but instead of facing psychiatrists and prescriptions, they are awarded with accolades and high paying salaries. These are people who are obsessed with success, or with the fear of failure, leading them to work compulsively. It may be the basketball player that has to make 20 free throws in a row before he can rest, or the investment banker that works through the night learning the minute details of a company's balance sheet. In my case, and the case of countless colleagues, it was an obsession with getting into medical school. After all, a large number of students enter college with the aspirations of becoming a doctor. It takes someone with the constant thoughts of being rejected from medical school and the need to succeed (the obsession), to motivate them enough to complete countless prerequisite courses, study for hours and hours for the MCAT, and meticulously complete countless, flawless applications for school (the compulsions). And even then, only a small fraction are accepted. This is the group that was the most compulsive. I remember taking a bathroom break in between sections during the MCAT, and in the bathroom was an Asian student holding some notes in one hand to cram before the next section, while urinating with the other hand. This is the world of the pre-med student. So it comes as no surprise that once you get to medical school and look around at your fellow classmates, you see people that were just as obsessed as you were about success. I will admit to locking myself in a library with lunch in hand and studying physiology for 18 straight hours. The scary thing is, I don't consider myself nearly as obsessive as many of my other classmates. One can only imagine what they put themselves through when it comes to studying.

I've learned that we all are obsessive-compulsive beings. It is merely the nature of our obsessions that separate the successful from the pathologic. Perhaps it's true when the famous composer and author Oscar Levant said, "There's a fine line between genius and insanity." I hope I've convinced you that this line may not even exist. And if you still aren't convinced we all have a bit of OCD, perhaps you missed something and should read this chapter again.

Chapter 16

Keeping a Healthy Distance

As a medical student, it is easy to get attached to patients. Since a student usually only follows two or three patients, we have time to get to know our patients better than anyone else on the team. This allows us time to meet the families, to hear their stories, and to get to know the person behind the diagnosis. Some may say that getting attached to patients is never a good idea, because one can't allow personal connections and emotions to factor into medical decision-making. Others would argue that this level of involvement is a wonderful thing, and this attachment is part of caring for patients. Coming into medical school, my mindset was more towards the latter. Thoughts of helping others were still fresh in my head.

But I came across two patients that pushed me a little more towards the "keep your distance" side of the equation.

The first case happened to be the very first patient I ever took care of as a student. To maintain patient confidentiality, let's call her DeeDee. She was a child who suffered from gastroschisis, a disease in which you are born with part of your intestines hanging outside of the abdomen through a hole in the abdominal wall. No one is exactly sure how this disease develops. The abdominal wall closes in from both sides when we are developing as fetuses inside the womb. For some reason, the wall does not form completely in children with gastroschisis, and the intestines (and even other organs like the liver) may stick out from the hole. It is no doubt a frightening sight when your child has parts of their intestines hanging out of the body. Luckily, the gut can usually be put back into place slowly over the first few days of life, and the hole in the abdomen can be easily fixed with stitches. Unfortunately, sometimes the gut has a hard time getting blood to parts that are outside of the belly, and therefore, pieces of the intestine die. These pieces have to be cut out, and the living parts reattached. Sadly for DeeDee, she was born with gastroschisis, and much of her bowel had died and had to be removed. She was left with short gut syndrome, a state where you don't have enough intestine to properly absorb enough nutrition. It's a devastating illness, because these kids have to receive nutrition directly into their blood stream. To do this, a central line must be placed, which is essentially a tube that is inserted through a large vein (often the subclavian vein, in the upper chest), and pushed through until the tip reaches into the heart. The other end of the tube is outside the body, where the nutrition can be given. Often, these kids don't live long, due to a combination of malnutrition and infections caused by bacteria entering the blood stream through the very line that keeps them alive.

DeeDee was in the hospital for the entire month I was on the pediatric inpatient rotation. Every morning, at 6AM, I would go into her room, and even though she was only 2, she knew the morning routine. She would roll over and lay on her side so I could listen to her heart and lungs. Later in the day, when I had free time, I would go in her room and play with the variety of toys she had lying around, and try to keep her entertained. Her mother had decided to give her up for adoption, fearing she could not take care of such a sick child. She rarely visited. All day in a crib with no parents around must have been torture, so I knew she enjoyed the time we spent together. Often when the team would walk by her room during rounds, we would hear her saying my name, or at least trying to say my name, hoping to get my attention to have another play session. My team thought it was rather cute, and I grew attached to her. She was, after all, my first patient.

My month of pediatrics came to an end, so I said goodbye to DeeDee. But only a few weeks later, she was transferred to a hospital that was closer to her family members. Well, this hospital happened to be in my hometown, and I soon found myself back home visiting my parents. So, I decided to surprise DeeDee and go visit her in the new hospital. With stuffed animal in hand, I went to the children's floor, and asked the nurses where I could find her. "She's right there," the nurse said, pointing to the corner. There was DeeDee, sitting in a chair next to the nurse's station, staring up at me. There was some hint of recognition in her eyes, but not exactly what I was expecting. The nurse and she went outside to play on the swings, so I accompanied them. DeeDee didn't say much to me, just went about her routine. So, after 10 minutes, I decided it was time to go back home, and left her with the stuffed animal. After one month of spending every day seeing her, it only took three weeks, and she had all but forgotten about me. She was only two, and there were obviously many members of the medical staff involved in her care, so it only made sense she didn't remember everyone. But to me, she was a special patient, maybe because she was my first patient, and maybe because I felt that I made a difference in her hospital stay. It sounds silly, but it did hurt a little when she didn't recognize me. Perhaps it would be better to not get attached to patients, I told myself.

The second patient encounter was during my final year of medical school, during a pediatric neurology rotation. We were consulted by the general pediatrics team to come evaluate a patient with headache and ataxia (which means difficulty walking and coordinating movement). He was a 9 year old, and it was obvious from the first glance that something was terribly wrong with him. His eyes were constantly moving rapidly from side to side. When he got up to go to the bathroom, his limbs moved in unsteady, jerking motions, and his own legs could barely support his weight. We asked him to touch our finger with his, then touch his nose, a test of coordination. It took him a few seconds to actually get his arm moving, as if he wanted to move it, but it just wouldn't move. And when it did, it flew out as if it was out of his control. We thought that he had likely developed an infection, and that the immune system had made antibodies to fight off the infection. Unfortunately, sometimes the body makes antibodies that also accidentally attack parts of the human body's own cells, known as auto-immune disease. For him, his antibodies were also attacking his brain. In essence, his brain was becoming inflamed from the attack of his body's antibodies. His brain was slowly losing more and more of its function. The attending pediatric neurologist said he had seen cases like this before, and they often get very sick before they get better, but luckily, they do usually get better.

Unfortunately, he kept getting sicker. By day 3, he couldn't walk at all, and within a week, he had slipped into a coma and had to be placed in the intensive care unit, where a breathing tube was placed to keep him alive. When the brain loses enough of its function, the parts that control breathing can also stop working, resulting in death unless artificial ventilation can be started, as was the case here. For the next three weeks, we would come into his room every day, and check various aspects of neurologic function, such as his reflexes and how his pupils responded to light. We would comment on the small changes that were happening from day to day, with no real progress, despite trying a variety of therapies such as steroids and plasmapheresis (which filters out many of the antibodies floating around in your blood), in hopes that if his body truly were attacking itself, this would get rid of some of the attackers. Progress was slow and on some days, non-existent. The parents were obviously distraught at having a son that was completely normal one minute, and now a step away from dying. Truly every parent's nightmare.

My month with pediatric neurology came to an end, and still he remained in the intensive care unit. I left, not knowing what would happen with him, but praying for the best. It was once again a case where I had become attached to a patient and a family over the course of the month.

Four months later, as I strolled through the lobby of the hospital on my way home, I saw a familiar face. It was his mother. My brain quickly tried to remember the context of how I knew her. When I realized who she was, the next question was how to go about asking about her son. After all, he may have died, or may be suffering from brain damage, or may still be in the intensive care unit in a coma. I had no idea. Hospital regulations forbade us from looking at patient records other than for those patients who we are directly involved with at the time, so as soon as I had left the pediatric neurology service, I did not look into his files to see what had happened. So, I posed the neutral question, "How is everything going?" Her face lit up, and she said everything was going well. She was just waiting for Cody to get out of the bathroom. They were in the hospital for a follow-up visit. My smile couldn't be contained.

"So he's fine?"

"Yes, back to his normal self."

And just then, out from the bathroom ran a Cody I had never seen before. Healthy, full of energy, and a normal 9 year old.

"Cody, oh my god, it's so good to see you." I felt like giving him a big bear hug, but tried to maintain my professional composure. He looked at me for a second, slightly perplexed. And then...

"Do I know you?"

In the one month I had been seeing Cody everyday, he had been in a coma. He had only seen me briefly when he was first admitted to the hospital before he got really sick. So, it came as no surprise that he had no idea who I was. It was awkward feeling so close to a person and caring so much about their well-being, and yet they have no idea who you are.

Both of these encounters left me wondering about the level of emotional investment we as physicians should make in our patients. There is an important balance between caring about patients, and being distant enough to protect your sanity when things go wrong or patient's die. But in the end, it seems that the rewards of medicine come from seeing those you care about get better, and that true care can only come when you are invested fully in your patients. Even if the patients forget you (or have no idea who you are), I still think we owe it to them to be emotionally invested in their well-being. And if at some point down the road that means becoming upset with the loss of a patient, that's okay.

Chapter 17

Awkward Moments

In 1966, an anthropologist named Edward Hall introduced the term proxemics. Proxemics is the study of spatial relationships between humans or other animals as they relate to various social contexts. Simply put, it is the study of personal space. For humans, when we interact with each other, there are social norms for how close you should be to another person, and based on your culture, social status, population density, and many other factors, each of us has some differences in what we consider appropriate. For the average American, it is thought that people begin feeling uncomfortable when someone is within 24 inches on each side, within 27 inches in front, or within about 16 inches behind them, excluding intimate relationships of course. In the doctor's office, there is a completely different set of social norms, one in which a doctor is allowed to enter the patient's personal space, and then examine, poke, prod, and listen to a patient's body. While this deviation from typical social norms is usually not considered the least bit unusual for a patient or experienced doctor, someone entering the medical field sees and feels it all too clear. Every doctor-in-training has to adjust to this newly found permission to enter the personal space of complete strangers. Listening to the heart, examining the abdomen, and looking into ears may seem routine, but for a new medical student, feelings of self-consciousness and inadequacy are the rule rather than the exception. But with practice, one develops a comfort level quickly with the routine exam. Soon the student is deftly moving from one part of the examine to the next with comfort and flow, holding instruments like a stethoscope and tongue depressor with a confident and steady hand. Unfortunately, there are a few areas of the examination that are not routine, and not as easy to develop a comfort with. Most medical schools provide focused learning sessions for these particular physical exam areas. For us, these came during our first and second year. Each particular session pushed the limits of what we were comfortable with, all in an attempt to teach us how to properly examine the human body and get acquainted with invading the most personal parts of a patient's personal space.

The first session was held by a group of women's health advocates. They went around and taught students the basics of the breast exam. That's right, this group would go from school to school and allow students to examine their breasts. We divided into groups of five or six, and unfortunately, I was placed in a group of all females, which only added to my sense of discomfort. The instructor gave us step-by-step instructions on how to position the patient, and how to properly examine the breasts. This involved walking our fingers over every inch of the breast and pressing down with different amounts of pressure to feel for any masses. When it was time to perform the exam, it became obvious that this technique took a painfully, awkwardly long time. As the exam started, thoughts were racing in my mind regarding the best way to stay cool and not appear uncomfortable. Usually when you are this close to a patient and examining them, you talk to them to break the tension. But what do you talk about when you're examining someone's breasts? "Lovely weather we're having." "How about those Mets?" Perhaps I would just keep my mouth shut. It was a little easier knowing this woman had her breasts examined all the time, and that this was not weird for her in the slightest. This fact made me more confident and less self-conscious. When my turn came, I stayed focused on the task, went about the exam just as they had taught, and kept the conversation to a minimum. Overall, I felt the whole experience went pretty smoothly. But there were plenty of my fellow students who I'm sure were crippled with nervousness during their turn. You can imagine the quiet, academic, shy student who has avoided having to deal with breasts by hiding in books his whole life. Medical school has a few of those. I'd pay good money to see him perform a breast exam.

So, the first of the awkward physical exam sessions was over. But the next would push the limits of uncomfortable encounters even further. Before our OBGYN rotation, we had to learn the female pelvic exam. I wasn't quite sure how this was going to work. Maybe they had mannequins or detailed anatomic models for us to practice with. We were divided up into small groups once again, and were assigned to one teacher. Ours was a middle-aged woman who spoke very eloquently, and in a straight-forward and didactic fashion, told us all about how to insert the speculum. This tool resembles a duck's closed bill, is inserted into the vagina, and then opened in order to view the cervix, which lies deep inside. We learned how to do a bimanual exam in which we feel for ovaries from inside the vagina. This was all very scary stuff. At the end of the teaching session, it was time to practice. Still, no mannequin in sight. She instructed us to step outside the room, and come in one at a time, and to pretend as if you were seeing an actual patient from beginning to end. She also said to give her a few minutes while she disrobed! Holy crap, we were going to be doing these pelvic exams on her! It was difficult to believe that someone would be willing to take on such a task. Each of the instructors must have had pretty strong beliefs in women's health and education to put up with this. I made my way into the room when it was my turn, and fumbled through the exam. I constantly asked her if she was doing okay throughout, both as a way of avoiding awkward silences, and to try to convince both her, and probably myself, that I wasn't nervous. In the end, the exam went fine, and there was a good deal of learning that came about as a result of the session. But there were still tons of questions floating around in my head regarding these instructors. One can't help but wonder if they're married and, if so, what their spouses think of this job. And how much does one get paid to be examined in this way by medical students? I'll probably never know, but I do wonder.

So, the tough exams were done, or so I thought. They saved the best for last. Rectal exams and the male genitals! Oh yes, there are groups of men who serve as teachers for these exams as well, and yes, we ended up performing the physical exam on them. They were all mostly older men, and our small group of students took turns sticking our fingers where no fingers should go. Our instructor got into three different positions and allowed us to try the exam in all three ways. That was a total of 15 rectal exams! Add this to the penile exam and the testicular exam, where we had to ram our fingers up into the testicles to feel for hernias, and it made for a rough day for the instructor. But once again, people did this, a job I thought no one would sign up for.

Looking back, there is probably no better way to learn these invasive exams than through these teaching sessions. How difficult would it be to perform the exam for the first time on an actual patient? But apart from the examination, I also learned that my previously established social norms for personal space no longer applied. I would have to adapt to this new set of rules. It was the first step in a long road to becoming comfortable with my future role as a doctor.

Chapter 18

Off With Their Heads

During our third year of medical school, our curriculum takes a unique turn. Most schools are organized so that students get two years of classroom education and two years in the hospital. Our school condenses two years in the classroom into one by simply teaching the basic materials. We do our two years of hospital training during our second and fourth years. But wait, you say, if you do only one year of classroom lectures whereas other schools do two, don't you learn half as much? Yes, one could argue this. However, the reality of medical school, and essentially all of classroom learning, is that we memorize enough to do well on the test, and then press the "delete" key in our brains to make room for material we have to memorize for our next exam.

None of us truly remembers the details of high school calculus, right? So really, one less year of memorizing and forgetting was fine by me.

So, we are left with a wide open third year, during which time we are let loose to explore research interests for the entire year. Whether it be sitting at a laboratory bench doing work in basic science, or collecting data on actual patients through clinical research, the year is wide open with possibility. And for those that aren't inclined to spend the year doing research, they are allowed to take the year and work towards a second degree.

For me, I decided to participate in basic science research. I spent the year working at a laboratory bench, exploring a very specific topic with hopes of discovering something new and being able to publish my findings in a scientific journal. I had already decided that pediatric neurology would be my future career, so I chose to work on epilepsy research. My goal was to study a particular part of the brain known as the hippocampus. This was the region of the brain which was thought to hold the key in understanding how we develop seizures. In order to study the brain and how it changes during seizures, we used the brains of mice. The year was very mind opening.

Working with animals is difficult. Personally, my opinion of animal testing in laboratories has been mixed.

On the one hand, it is unfair for us humans to take advantage of helpless animals and use them for our own gains in medicine. On the other hand, there are people suffering from diseases which we can potentially treat one day, and animal studies often provide useful data to help unlock clues to future treatment. Isn't it better to do experiments on animals instead of on humans?

To start our research, we walked over to a nearby building which held all of the research animals. We would pick out a group of mice for an experiment, and cover their cages with sheets when walking out of the building so as not to anger any animal activists that may be walking by. The mice were then given injections that caused them to start seizing. Once they seized for long enough, they were given injections to stop the seizure. If they survived this process, their brains had to be collected to evaluate for changes. This is where it got tricky, and disgusting. To make this humane, the mice were injected with ketamine, a chemical which would prevent them from feeling any pain. Once we thought they were sufficiently doped up, I had to place the mice one at a time into what is best described as a tiny guillotine. But instead of a blade falling down, I had what was essentially one of those paper cutters we used in elementary school to cut large pieces of paper. So down came the blade, severing the mouse's head. When the blade was dull, this would take two or three gruesome swings of the blade. And the most difficult part was sometimes watching the headless body start jumping and twitching as impulses from the severed spinal cord were sent shooting through the body. Even the severed head would sometimes move, as the muscles in the head contracted for one last time. It was horrendous. But as soon as the head was chopped off, it was immediately stuck into liquid nitrogen in order to freeze the brain, thereby preventing further damage to brain tissue from lack of oxygen. I then had to cut open the head and delicately remove the brain, hopefully intact. I must have cut off the heads of 100 mice during my year. I hated doing it every time, and kept justifying it with the hopes that my work would someday help patients.

But not all of the work was this gruesome. Eventually, once the grunt work was done, I began to look at one particular structure in the neurons of these mice known as actin, which I hypothesized played a role in epilepsy in a location of the brain called the hippocampus. Actin is the skeleton of the neuron, helping it keep its shape. It was a structure no one had looked at before in epilepsy. There was a chemical that was used to beautifully stain molecules of actin, and I stained lots of brain slices in hopes of seeing a difference between mice with seizures and normal mice. I never thought this type of thing could get me excited, but one evening, late in the lab, I had just stained a large number of slides, and was about to look under the microscope for the first time. It was then that I realized I was likely the only person in the world to look at this particular part of the brain, at this particular structure, in this particular disease. This would be a peak into the mystery of how we are made, the very goal of research. As I loaded the slides into the microscope, I could actually feel my heart pounding. And lo and behold, there was truly a difference between the normal mice and ones that were seizing! It was amazing.

The tough thing about basic science research is that in order to truly claim a new discovery, you have to prove you've found something with lots of different experiments. Unfortunately, I could not replicate my results with other experiments, and therefore, could not share my findings with the world through a publication in a science journal. Yet, I know this was something significant, and am sure someone will prove it someday.

All in all, it was an amazing year in the lab. I realized I lacked the patience to do this type of research my whole life, but gained an admiration for those that dedicate their lives to the lab in hopes of advancing our field.

Chapter 19

Every Student's Enemy

There is a voice that constantly speaks to you. The voice pops up at the most inconvenient times. It brings up past failures, and weighs you down with pessimism. The voice follows you every moment of the day, and is impossible to avoid. This voice is the self-conscious of the medical student. For some, the voice speaks much louder than for others, and for the ones fortunate enough to have a quiet self-conscious, medical school becomes much easier. But every student has this voice, and it can become a true burden for some.

The simple fact of medical school is that you end up throwing together a bunch of over-achievers, those that excelled during their undergraduate years and were at the top of the class. But all of the sudden, they are placed into an environment where everyone is bright, and they become simply "average". The change from superstar to mediocre leads to a great deal of self-doubt for the typical student. No one really talks about these feelings, but it happens to everyone.

Take myself for example. There were multiple times during my first year where I worked relentlessly to learn the minutia of basic science. But when it came time for the exam, I would end up doing only average. "How did they do it?" I'd ask myself of those that were at the top of the class. After all, I was working constantly, so how did they know more than I did?

We would have smaller group discussions a few times a week in which we would discuss topics with a professor. The 15 or so students would go over the material and ask questions. Every now and then, the professor would throw out questions to the group, and for the majority of these questions, I had no idea what the answer was. But someone in the lab always knew the answer. And with every answer I didn't know and someone else did, I felt progressively more stupid.

Given the fact I felt this way, I can only imagine how those that were doing worse than the average felt. The medical student brain does not accept average, and below average is usually not even on the radar, but someone in medical school has to be below average. In fact, half of us have to be below average.

I eventually developed ways to come to terms with the voice in my head telling me that I wasn't cut out for a life in medicine. For example, sitting in lab, I realized I was putting myself up against the entire lab. If I didn't know the answer to the question, and someone else did, that did not mean everyone knew the answer. Chances are, the majority of my classmates also didn't know the answer. And there were obviously a few times I knew the answer when no one else did. Everyone was in fact probably on very similar levels, but by placing myself against the entire lab, it was easy to make myself feel inadequate.

When all was said and done, I found myself in the upper 25% of my class. I have no doubt that even those that ended up in the top 10% doubted themselves on multiple occasions during medical school. It's a completely normal part of being in a competitive atmosphere. But I learned the importance of doing things at my own pace, and trying to focus on the finish line rather than on the other racers.

Chapter 20

The Anatomy Lab

The popular media has an interesting perception of the anatomy lab. Dissecting the human body is glorified as some kind of right of passage for a medical student. It weeds out the weak ones that can't handle the gore and blood, right? Well, not exactly.

We began work in the anatomy lab just a few months into our first year of medical school. Our entire class was divided into smaller groups so that there were six students for each cadaver. Before our work in the lab began, we had a session with our professors to get us geared up for the months ahead. The lecturers spoke philosophically about spirituality and the questions about our own mortality that would eventually arise by working with cadavers. They discussed the privilege we had as medical students to see the human body in such a unique way. This session probably made me even more nervous about what was ahead for us.

The first day arrived, and we hit the locker room to change into scrubs. As we entered the lab itself, there was an eerie quiet, with tables stretched in every direction, on top of which lay the bodies wrapped in large, black plastic sheets. Everyone knew what was underneath, but it's as if no one wanted to believe it until they actually saw it. We gathered around the table and were asked to uncover the cadaver. Ours was a slightly obese woman who was likely in her mid 50s, younger than most of the other cadavers. She looked fake at first, like a giant plastic doll, with a pale color and blank stare. But as we uncovered more of her, and saw her arms, her legs, all the parts constructed so precisely, so intricately, she soon became very real.

It's hard cutting into a cadaver for the first time. We stood around, read over our instruction manual a few times to ensure we were cutting in the right place, and then I eventually volunteered to make the first cut. Might as well try to be bold, or at least pretend to be, I thought. I gripped the scalpel tightly, and moved slowly, not wanting to make a mistake. My hand trembled slightly, but inside, it felt as if it was shaking uncontrollably. My hand came to a rest on her skin, steadying it. I put the scalpel to her skin for the first time, and began pressing down gently to begin my incision. Suddenly, she bolted upright and let out a blood curdling scream! Well, in my mind she did, but I tried to brush those images aside. The skin was tougher than I had thought it would be, and I found myself really working hard to cut through it. But eventually I made it through, and the most difficult cut of the entire month was over. We made small jokes throughout this first day, which were all quickly followed by nervous laughter. This became our lab group's defense mechanism of sorts. It was a way for us to get through the dissection without constantly thinking about the fact that we were cutting into another human. But despite this, every now and then, there were times of reflection, when thoughts about our cadaver drifted from the dissection to questions about her life. Was she a mother? What kinds of food did she like? Did she wonder what students would be dissecting her after she died? Would she have been happy with the way we were treating her? What would her family members think? What was her name? These human questions made it more difficult to cut into her day after day. The more difficult it was, the more we would laugh.

There were days that were particularly difficult, one of which was dissecting the hand. Maybe it's the uniquely human features of the hand that made it so difficult. We would pull on the tendons of the wrist and watch the fingers bend, giving motion to the lifeless body. It was amazing to see how a truly human action can be broken down into simple mechanics.

Another difficult day for me was dissecting out the brain. The first part involved removing the skull from the top of the head. We cut around the head with a buzzsaw. When we finally got all the way around, the skull was ready to be lifted off. It was as if we had cracked the lock on an ancient treasure chest, and would now see the riches inside. And there it was, the center of human life as we know it, the brain. We delicately cut the spinal cord attached to the bottom and all the various nerves attached to it. The brain was eventually completely loose. I pulled it out of the bony skull where it had faithfully resided for the past 50 years. I held it for a few seconds. There, in my hand, was the entire existence of this person. All of the memories of a lifetime, all of the knowledge, all of the love and emotions that made her who she was, all within this small object. The most advanced computer system ever built, and I could hold it in the palm of my hand. Unbelievable.

I don't consider myself a spiritual person. All of the classes that taught of the biology behind life, of

113

evolution, and of the basic science behind our universe made me question the existence of a higher being. But ironically, in this anatomy lab, a place one would imagine as the epitome of hard science, I found myself thinking more spiritually than ever before. With each dissection came more fascination with the wondrous and intricate construction of the human body. Every muscle, from the large muscles of the legs to the small muscles of the eye, lay in the exact same place in every cadaver. Each kidney, with millions of tiny threadlike nephrons, had at one point relentlessly worked to filter blood. Each brain, with its billions of neurons and hundreds of nerves that connected it to the rest of the body, lay in perfect harmony to create a beautiful network to control every process of the body. I couldn't help but think that such a perfect creation could only have come about through the work of a higher being. It was just too perfect.

The anatomy lab was undoubtedly a challenge. But no one dropped out of school because they couldn't deal with dissecting cadavers. No one fainted. No one vomited because of the gore. It was in no way a right of passage, but truly a privilege. For the first time, it became obvious that the field of medicine would allow me and my colleagues to see the human body in a way not many others ever would. And by getting this intimate look into the structure of the human body, we not only learned anatomy, but learned to appreciate the intricacies and precision within the human body. Along with this came the humbling realization that not even a lifetime of work as a physician would allow us time to learn about all of the body's complexities.

Chapter 21
The Match

Over 100 fourth year medical students sit together in a fancy conference room. They are surrounded by friends, family, and hospital faculty. On each table sits fancy hors-de-voirs, glasses filled with punch, and envelopes. The students whisper to one another and have smiles on their faces which attempt to mask an obvious uneasiness. One by one, each student is called to the front to pick up his/her envelope. Students nervously eye the envelope, some twirl it around their fingers, others hold it up to the light in a futile attempt to see what is written inside. Their anxiety is well-founded, because the letter inside these envelopes will determine how often they can see their families. It will separate friends and lovers and create new relationships. It will determine how students will spend much of their remaining years of youth.

It is Match Day, and inside the envelopes are the names of the hospitals where the students will start their residencies in a few short months. Without much exception, you go where it tells you to go, case closed. At this point, you've put yourself at the mercy of the match process.

The process of getting into a residency program is like no process any student has ever experienced before. During high school, students apply to multiple undergraduate institutions, get replies from these institutions, and if accepted to multiple places, have the opportunity to decide which institution to attend. The same applies to medical school. But getting into residency is a completely different beast.

It all starts off with a common application that the student sends to as many residency programs as he or she desires. The student is then invited to interview with the programs that deem them qualified for a spot in their residency program. After the interview is complete, the students must turn in a "rank list". This list consists of the programs at which the student interviewed, ranked in order of places the student would most like to go. This list is submitted electronically, and the residency programs submit similar lists of the students they interviewed, ranked according to who they considered most qualified. The computer system then takes every student list, and determines if their top ranked residency program also chose them to be part of the program. If so, the student matches at this program. If not, the computer moves to the next residency program on the student's list and determines if this institution ranked the student high enough to offer them a spot. The residency programs only have a set number of spots. Some subspecialized programs, such as neurosurgery or dermatology, may only have 2 or 3 spots available in their institution, whereas pediatrics and medicine tend to have many more, sometimes as many as 40 to 50 spots, depending on the size of the hospital.

Everyone in the country finds out where they matched on the same day, appropriately deemed "Match Day". It occurs in March during the last year of school, and there is typically a fancy ceremony in which everyone gets an envelope that contains the place they matched. At my school, everyone opens their envelopes at the same time, which leads to quite the spectacle as many people rejoice at matching at the program they ranked first, whereas others quietly leave the room and cry when they find out they matched at the program they ranked 6th, at an institution they really didn't want to attend. Residents could spend anywhere from three to seven years in this hospital, depending on the type of doctor they intend to become.

So what happens to the people that don't match at any of the programs on their rank list? A few days before Match Day, they get the dreaded e-mail which tells them they haven't matched anywhere, and a process known as "The Scramble" begins. These students work with their school's dean to get in touch with residency programs that didn't fill all of their open spots. The programs and students find one another, and thus, almost everyone ends up with a spot for match day. It's obviously stressful for the student to scramble, since they have to decide on a place to spend the next 3+ years of their lives, and they have to decide quickly, usually in the course of a day, since the unfilled spots fill up quickly.

The match day itself is obviously stressful, because even though you know you have matched, you are not sure where (unless you had to scramble). I've always felt that opening these envelopes in front of your peers is somewhat cruel. It forces people who didn't match at their top choice to put on a happy face for the crowd, and pretend that all is well. No one wants to let others know they didn't match where they wanted to go. After all, we hate to admit failure of any kind. Some schools go one step further on the cruel and unusual ladder and actually have students go up in front of the entire class and one by one, they open their envelopes and announce where they matched. How traumatic would it be to open the envelope and find out you'll be spending the next 5 years in Cold-as-crap, North Dakota at the program you ranked last. It's hard to cover up the disappointment.

I quickly learned that a life in medicine is a life of jumping through hoops, and the hoops never seem to end. The match process is just one of these hoops.

Chapter 22

Seizures and Pools Don't Mix

In October of 1825, a young man entered the University of Edinburgh Medical School in England. His intent was to pursue the field of medicine, as his father had. But he found the study of medicine dull and unappealing. His fascination laid in geology, and the study of life. It was not long before he set off on a five year voyage around the world that would change the course of history. On this journey, he put together a fascinating record of species the world had never before seen. The man was Charles Darwin, and the knowledge and observations made during this expedition led to the modern theory of natural selection. His theory was stated in the introduction of his work:

"As many more individuals of each species are born than can possibly survive; and as, consequently, there is a frequently recurring struggle for existence, it follows that any being, if it vary however slightly in any manner profitable to itself, under the complex and sometimes varying conditions of life, will have a better chance of surviving, and thus be *naturally selected*. From the strong principle of inheritance, any selected variety will tend to propagate its new and modified form."

-Charles Darwin, *On the Origin of Species,* 1859.

The concept was simple…those that have favorable traits are able to survive and produce offspring. Over time, the population has more members with these traits. New species are formed when old species move to new regions where a whole new set of traits now have the advantage, or if the environment itself changes.

In college, I would think about this concept, and wonder whether it applied to humans. Are we still evolving? Is there a trait that has some genetic basis that would be considered advantageous, thereby slowly changing the makeup of the human species over hundreds and thousands of generations? My conclusion was that we were evolving, but not in the old Darwinian sense where those that are more physically capable survive. We now lived in an environment where we did not have any predators, and for the most part, despite any physical disadvantages, you still had access to the food and water necessary to ensure survival and future reproduction. My theory was that we were slowly becoming smarter. After all, those that were more intelligent were able to obtain jobs with higher income. With this income, they could provide themselves with healthcare when they were sick, eat healthier diets, and have access to recreational facilities to ensure a healthy lifestyle. Intelligent people were more likely to avoid situations that endangered their well-being, such as using illicit drugs, driving intoxicated, or speeding down the freeway on their motorcycle without a helmet. And finally, smart people were more likely to protect their offspring from danger. They could install car seats correctly, afford vaccines, and have the resources to provide for more children. Sure each of these things may only affect someone's chances of survival by a very small fraction, but over thousands of generations, this would make a large difference, just as Darwin had observed with various other species.

My pediatric neurology rotation during the fourth year of medical school quickly debunked my theory. During this rotation, we often saw patients that suffered from seizure disorders. Seizures are events characterized by synchronous firing of neurons in our brains that lead the body to do very different things. Most people think of seizures as events where the person collapses and starts shaking uncontrollably, as if possessed by demons. But in actuality, seizures are very diverse, and can present in a variety of ways. For example, if the neurons that control the arm start firing together, the arm starts jerking uncontrollably. If they occur in brain areas that control eye movement, you'll often see someone with eyes that are stuck in one direction. Rare seizures that occur in areas that detect smell will manifest as funny odors to the patient. In short, a seizure can mimic anything the brain is capable of doing during its normal function. Often times, the firing of neurons will spread throughout the brain, leading to firing in multiple areas of the brain and causing what is known as a generalized seizure. These are the seizures we see on television in which the person loses consciousness and jerks uncontrollably.

Luckily for patients that suffer from seizure disorders, there are medicines that often times will completely prevent seizures. But unfortunately for some, no amount of medication can completely get rid of their seizures. During a day in the pediatric neurology clinic, I met one such patient. She was a young girl, probably 7 or 8 years old, who came in wearing a helmet. This is a bad sign in pediatric neurology. It means that the seizures are occurring so frequently that the patient needs a helmet to protect her head when she collapses from a seizure. This patient was indeed having seizures multiple times each week. During the visit, the doctor discussed changing some medications to help with control. Near the end of the visit, when the mother was almost out the door, she turned and very casually said,

"Oh, we're planning on getting a pool this month."

"A what?" the doctor asked, hoping the mother didn't say what he thought she said.

"A pool. It's getting hot outside, so the family wants a pool."

A pool for a patient with seizures is like a hemophiliac taking up knife juggling as a hobby. Any way you slice it, not a good idea. All it takes is one seizure in the pool with no one around to kill this child. So, the doctor calmly replied,

"That's definitely not a good idea, given your daughter's seizures."

"Well, it's going to be one of those pools that sits above the ground, so she can't really fall in."

"Still not a good idea."

The mother was obviously looking for approval from the doctor for this pool, but was not going to get it. I couldn't believe they would even consider it. I truly wanted to grab the woman and just shake her. But alas, shaking people is looked down upon in medical school, and even after.

So the patient left, saying they'd think more about it, but it seemed like she was pretty set on the idea. Rather unfortunate for the daughter she was supposedly caring for.

So far, my theory of human evolution seemed on target. It only seemed logical that such a parent would have a lower probability of having her genes continually passed on. But there was one problem with my theory...sheer numbers! This mother had five children. Surely, her genes would live on for generations to come. In fact, she would go on to have more descendents than almost anyone else I know, due to the simple fact she was spitting out lots of children.

In a world where Darwin's theory of natural selection does not apply to humans, we will undoubtedly stop evolving into more fit, more adapted creatures. Our gene pool will begin to favor those that can simply produce the largest quantity of descendants, not necessarily the most fit. Sadly, this could mean that we are indeed evolving, just in the wrong direction.

Chapter 23

A New Flavor of Chip

The anatomy lab was a constant stimulation to the senses. We would see the inner workings of the human body. We would hear lectures from leading anatomists. The smell of the formalin-preserved cadavers would flood our noses every time we stepped into the lab. And we would feel the bones, the muscles, and the organs of our cadaver as we dissected further and further. All the senses were covered...almost.

Potato chips were one of my staples during lunch break. On one occasion, I had only gotten halfway through a bag, and the rest was left unfinished, tucked away in my bookbag, and forgotten about. For three hours every other day, the bookbag was left in the locker room of the anatomy lab.

Two weeks later, while studying in the library, I came across this bag of uneaten potato chips. It's a good feeling when you find food unexpectedly. After the first bite of the potato chips, there was a funny taste, something that was somewhat familiar, but I couldn't quite place it. Maybe they are just a little stale, I thought, but kept eating. A few of my fellow classmates soon walked in and joined my table. Being the nice person that I am, my potato chips were placed in the middle of the table as a communal offering. One of them took the offer, and began eating a chip. He stopped mid bite, a look of horror and disgust filled his face.

"These chips taste like dead people!"
Ahh yes, so that was the familiar taste. The smell of the formalin preservative from the anatomy lab had set into my chips. The chips were left unfinished. A lesson learned – the anatomy lab lockers were not a place to store food, and when it comes to chips, stick with the BBQ flavor.

Chapter 24

The First Patient

During our very first year of medical school, we would participate in what was known as the Practice Course for half a day each week. This was a class in which we would learn the art of medicine, such as how to interview patients, ways to build rapport, etc. As part of the course, during the end of our first year, we were set up with a doctor to follow around clinic a half day each week to see medicine in action. It was entertaining to just sit back, listen and watch how they did business. Then, about one month into this clinical experience, after a morning of seeing patients together, the doctor turned to me, handed me a chart, and said,

"Why don't you go see this patient?"

"On my own you mean?" I asked nervously.

"Yes, this one is all yours."

My heart began racing. I had to walk into a room on my own and try to help this patient. The chart said it was a teenager who had a fever and cold symptoms for two days. What should I ask her? What should we do for her? Would she ask me questions? What would I say? All these thoughts raced through my head as I knocked lightly on the door and walked in. Inside sat the teenage girl and her mother. The girl was on the examining table, and she was crying. Apparently, she felt miserable. After trying to comfort her, I made attempts to ask questions, but the girl continued to sob and ignored me. The mother was of little help, and made a few weak attempts to convince her daughter to listen to my questions. After a few minutes of fumbling around with random questions, I realized I was not getting anywhere. I was scared to even try examining her for fear the crying would worsen, so I just left the room.

Outside I found the attending physician, and explained the situation, conveying the information I had gotten during my short interview, which was minimal at best. He gave a slight understanding smile, and we went in together to finish up the visit.

Looking back on this visit, it's amazing how far a student comes during the course of medical school. Near the end of my four years, knocking on patient doors and walking in to get their stories came naturally, and there was no hesitation. No matter what awaited me behind the door, there was a sense of comfort with the amount of knowledge I had, and knowing that by the end of the visit, I would have some sense of what was causing the problem, and that if the patient had questions, I would at least be able to give some educated answers.

No matter what makes us nervous in life, it's feeling prepared that gets us through it. Whether it be preparing for a large presentation, or studying for a board exam, the more you know, the less nervous you become. Hopefully, dealing with patients will continue to get easier and easier through residency and beyond.

Chapter 25
The Bad News

When a patient comes into the hospital, something in the body has gone wrong. If all goes well, the patient will make a full recovery, and they will go home no worse for the wear. But this is often not the case, and in the worst case scenarios, the patient will not make it out of the hospital alive. When the inevitable becomes clear to doctors, the next step is conveying this to the patient. Giving a patient bad news is one of the most difficult parts of medicine. The way a doctor delivers the news often distinguishes the good doctors from the great ones.

The first time I had to witness this conversation, it was difficult. We were in the VA Hospital, short for Veteran's Affairs. The hospital was right across the street from the main hospital, and cared for those that had served in the armed forces for our country. It was one of the benefits they received for their service. This was where I met a man in his mid 60's that had been diagnosed with liver failure secondary to chronic hepatitis B infection. He had gotten the infection through a blood transfusion he received when he was younger after being shot during a bar fight. When your liver starts failing, blood flowing through it can often slow down, and blood starts backing up in all the veins that drain into the liver. Additionally, your liver makes protein that floats in your blood and helps keep fluid in your vessels. So, in liver failure, fluid starts leaking out of your engorged veins and pools up in places like your abdomen. His belly was huge, and he came in because he was having difficulty breathing with all the fluid that had built up, and needed some removed. This was done by placing a needle into his belly and draining the excess fluid. We removed close to two liters, and although he still had a great deal of fluid left, pulling more than this at once could have been dangerous for his health. The body is not used to having such large amounts of fluid added or removed at once. Later in his stay, we decided to do some imaging studies of his liver to assess for cancer, sometimes a result of chronic hepatitis infection. The results of our CT scan shocked us. This man had a clot going all the way from his liver, through the vein that connects to his heart, and down into the inside of his heart, where it was flapping around with each heart beat. This was bad news for him. Any minute the large clot could break off and go straight into his lungs, leading to a quick death. Sadly, there was not much we could do for him. When we went to tell him the news, he was obviously distraught, but not all that surprised.

"Well, can't I get a liver transplant or something?" he asked, trying desperately to look for a possible solution to his condition.

"Unfortunately, at this point, you would not be a candidate for a liver transplant," the resident told him matter-of-factly, but still with a touch of sympathy.

The patient nodded, almost to himself, and sat back in his bed. I couldn't make eye contact with him, I felt so bad. What must it feel like to hear that your life will soon be coming to an end. Everything you knew, everything you worked for, everyone around you would soon be gone. It was hard to imagine. We left to give him some time to think and come up with questions.

I came back later to speak with him some more. Like many VA patients, he did not have any family with him. He didn't quite understand what was happening, and asked me if I could explain what the situation was. So, taking out a pen and paper, I began drawing a diagram of the liver and heart, explaining where this clot was, and how large it was. He attempted to follow along for a while, but then eventually told me not to worry about it. He had resigned himself to his fate, and must have decided he didn't need to know the details. As I was leaving, he looked at me and thanked me for my help. I looked back and thanked him for all he had done for us. After all, he had risked his life in the Vietnam War fighting on behalf of this country. He appreciated the acknowledgement.

"I don't often hear that, thanks," he said.

It was always so ironic to me that a man who had survived one of the bloodiest wars of all time was now on his death bed because he got shot in a bar fight. It seemed cruel and unfair. Yet even though he was nearing the end of his life, he appreciated the care he was receiving, and part of it was likely because of the way he was told of his fate – with compassion, sympathy, and a listening ear. He knew we cared about him, and in a sense, that was all he needed. He needed to know that all had been done for him.

In the end, I learned that giving bad news doesn't necessarily have to be a negative experience for the doctor or patient. The important thing is that when you tell them, you give them a glimpse of how you are feeling as well.

Patients know when you care, and they come to accept bad news much easier if they know you're with them through their struggle.

Chapter 26

Those Three Little Words

The very last rotation of second year was internal medicine. It is perhaps the most mentally challenging of all the core rotations. Here, they take care of pretty much any adult health problem that does not involve surgery. Pneumonia, heart failure, kidney disease, pacreatitis...they see it all. Of the two months dedicated to this rotation, my entire second month was spent across the street from Duke at the VA Hospital. This was a government-run hospital, and the building was a huge brick eye sore. The colossal building was staffed by residents and attendings from Duke. This worked out well, since the hospital benefited from having a constant pool of workers from right across the street, and Duke had another facility in which to train residents and employ physicians. It also worked out well for physicians who were well past retirement age but still wanted to work. You see, Duke had a policy by which anyone aged 75 had to automatically retire, without exception. This avoided the awkward task of having to kick out those that would become a liability rather than an asset in their old age, as often happens when physicians age and can't keep up with the latest advances in medicine. However, the VA had no such policy. And as you can imagine, there are some doctors that are still as sharp as tacks, even at 75, and after a lifetime of building their medical knowledge, have no desire to stop working and take up shuffleboard. Dr. Steele was one of those doctors.

Dr. Steele (whose name I've changed, more to protect myself than him) was a veteran himself. It was obvious he was high ranking in his service, because he ran a tight ship. There was no give to him. He was a medium height and build, with hair that had completely grayed, and a face that did not have a trace of softness. His expression was always stern, and his words succinct and pointed. And when he talked, you listened. He would walk into the room in the morning and not have to say a word, as the room would get quiet and everyone would begin taking seats to start rounding. He ran things a bit different, as each morning we would sit and talk about every patient as a group, then walk around and see everyone. He would approach patients with a style that left no doubt who was in charge. He would matter-of-factly state his intention to examine the patient. If they attempted to talk, he would stop them, and inform them they could talk after he was done with his exam. It was clear he was the product of an age of medicine in which the hierarchy was even more defined and the doctor was always right.

As one can probably imagine, presenting patients to this man was no picnic. It was a constant test of fortitude. Every patient we presented would trigger countless, pointed questions to test our knowledge of both medicine and our patients. It was not a friendly manner in which he went about asking those questions, but one instead that made you feel as if you were in the spotlight in front of an audience, being asked to recite lines you hadn't time to memorize. And if the answer was incorrect, he would stop you mid-sentence with a, "No, that is wrong," and with no show of sympathy, would go into a long discussion of the answer. This would be followed by yet another, more difficult question. And since you didn't know the answer to the first one, this next answer would no doubt be incorrect as well. It was an uncomfortable exchange. Although he did attempt to teach, he did not fit "the teacher" description of pimping as we discussed before, because I don't think teaching was his only motive. He wanted to break us.

Sadly, with one resident on our team, he succeeded. This resident was in the family medicine residency, and they rotate through a variety of specialties during their training, one of which is internal medicine. Whether it's fair or not, different residency programs get different amounts of respect based on how competitive of a field it is. Family medicine is considered by many to be the least competitive field to get into, and therefore, people in this field are incorrectly labeled as less intelligent than those in other fields. However, this particular resident was not up to par, and Dr. Steele could sense this weakness. Like a deer lost from her herd, the resident would timidly begin her presentation, and Dr. Steele would eye her down, slowly approach while she was not looking, and pounce! I dreaded the moment each morning when she would have to present, because I knew questions were coming, and I knew she would not be able to answer them. Dr. Steele would add insult to injury by often showing a look of surprise when she did not know the answer. The added tension of him being an old Caucasian male and her being a young African American female led me to feel even more uncomfortable as this same routine played out

141

day after day. What's worse is that the resident was truly making an effort, but even when she would get some questions correct, Dr. Steele would simply ask harder questions. Halfway through the rotation, I noticed that the other residents were putting in orders on her patients. Dr. Steele had taken away her privileges to put in orders, stating he was worried about patient safety. This was something I had never seen done to a resident. To a doctor-in-training, such a loss is soul crushing. She left the rotation early, stating she had other obligations. The real reason she left was clear; he had broken her.

By now you understand the person we were up against. So, was I trembling in my boots every morning when it was my turn to present? Would I be his next victim? Did I stay awake at night, fearing my next embarrassing encounter with him? No. Why? Because in my corner I had those three little words. These three little words would disarm him of his ability to intimidate and embarrass. I would use them over and over again.

I take you back one year to the very start of my second year of medical school, when we started rotations. The art of pimping was new to me. Having to answer questions from people smarter than you in front of everyone on the team was uncomfortable. Students handle these questions in a variety of ways, just as physicians "pimp" us in different ways. Allow me to introduce you to some of the more common styles of responding to being pimped:

1. The Rambler – this student will answer each question with a verbal diarrhea of sorts, saying everything he knows about the topic in a muffled voice in hopes that the attending will hear one or two key words and declare his answer correct.

Attending: "Tell me about triple therapy for reflux."

Student: "Sure, reflux is something we see quite frequently in our adult population of patients. The treatments are quite varied, and triple therapy is one option amongst many. Ramble, ramble, ramble, antacids, ramble, ramble, infection, ramble, ramble."

Attending: "That's right, we use triple therapy for H. pylori infections."

Student: (to himself) Whew, that was close.

2. The Egotist – Comparatively, smarter than his fellow students. Takes on each question with an air of unfaltering confidence, with the misperception that acting as if he knows something will convince people that he actually knows something. He argues with anyone that tries to correct him, even the attending. Even when he's wrong,

you almost want to believe he is right, just because of the confidence. These people go on to become surgeons.

Attending: "This patient just had his second seizure in the setting of a fever, what would you do next?"

Student: "He needs a CT scan and a lumbar puncture."

Attending: "Well, he's three years old, and his neurologic exam is normal. He looks great right now, so there is no need for either."

Student: "But you don't want to miss a big tumor or something."

Attending: "With a normal exam, that's not likely."

Student: "Well this could be the start of a meningitis."

Attending: "He would not look so well on exam. Besides, the guidelines say he doesn't need it."

Student: "You can't always go by guidelines. What if this kid dies?"

Attending: "Let's move on."

Student: (to himself) Everyone's an idiot, except me.

3. The Nervous Deflector – each question is met by a nervous shuffle through papers, a few "um's" and "uh's", and an attempt to scan the floor in hopes that the answer is magically written on the tiles. This student finishes by nervously glancing at someone else in the group, thereby deflecting the question to this new person with a visual

"tag, you're it." The attending turns towards this new person, and the Nervous Deflector is off the hook. Get a few of these in your group, and the question bounces from person to person through glance after glance, until the attending finally gives up and answers his own question. These students go on to become pathologists, who stare at specimens on slides all day and avoid human contact.

4. The Tangentialist – If the answer is not known, the student will simply state something she does know that somehow relates to the topic.
Attending: "What antibiotic would you use in this patient?"
Student: "Well, the rate of resistant bacteria is becoming a big problem in the community."
Attending: "That's true. In this case, I'd probably go with vancomycin."
Student: "Yeah, that's what I was thinking."

5. The Name-Dropping Data Collector – This student remembers a variety of recent studies, recalls the name of the physician that wrote the studies, and uses them when the moment is right. These people go into internal medicine.

145

Attending: "What organism do you think is causing this patient's pneumonia?"

Student: "Well, the internal medicine chairman, Dr. Holmes, recently put out a study that says the rate of strep pneumonia infections are highest for this county."

Attending: (trying not to refute his own chairman) "Uh, yeh, that's right."

6. The Generalist – Uses a sequence of progressively more and more general statements without ever really answering the question. They make no definitive statements. These students become radiologists.

Attending: "What is the first line drug for hypertension?"

Student: "Well, I don't think our hospital has a set algorithm for that."

Attending: "Actually, we do."

Student: "Right, but what I'm saying is that there is no good data on this question."

Attending: "Actually, there is."

Student: "Well, every patient is different."

7. The Combinator – Combines the various strategies into one big attempt to save face.

Attending: "What do you think led to this new mutation in our patient's DNA?"

Student: "Well, Watson and Crick first described the structure of DNA."

Attending: "True, but that's not the question."

Student: "Dr. Holmes told us in a lecture that…"

Attending: (cutting the student off) "I don't want to know what Dr. Holmes thinks, I'm asking you."

Student: (Nervously glances at fellow student, who nervously glances back at him)

Attending: "Well?"

Student: "Uh, ramble, ramble, ramble, smoking, ramble."

Attending: "What did you say?"

Student: "Well, every patient is different."

As I began on the wards, I had no good strategy. I tried my hand as the Tangentialist, the Generalist, and even took a stab as the Egotist. But I never really felt comfortable. I knew I needed something else, a fail-safe resource I could rely on to avoid the nervousness, the pressure. Ideally, something I could program into a handheld device that would have all the answers. But sadly, there was no such thing. But one day near the beginning of second year, I had an epiphany. Something that was so simple, I couldn't believe more people didn't use it. All I needed were those three little words. So the next day, I decided to try it.

I could feel myself already less stressed as rounds began. A few questions were lobbed my way, but I knew the answer. Finally, the attending threw me a question that was tough, giving me a chance to use my weapon. I looked him straight in the eye, and without the slightest bit of hesitation, I let it out,

"I don't know."

And just as quick as I said it, the attending simply began teaching about the topic, educating us all. No nervous rambling, no glances at my fellow students for help, just those three words and I was out of the spotlight.

But wait you say, aren't you losing points because you are admitting you don't know? Well, I'm convinced that a confident "I don't know" makes you look much smarter than nervously stumbling over the answer. In time, I would tweak my "I don't know" so that I said it not only confidently, but with a tone that made me sound almost a bit surprised that I didn't know the answer, thereby giving off the impression that I knew everything else except the answer to that particular question. Of course, for this strategy to work, you do have to correctly answer some questions, or risk people catching on.

I eventually learned that not knowing isn't the end of the world. No one is expected to know everything, especially medical students. After all, if I already knew everything I wouldn't be paying $50,000 a year to be in school. It's a lesson I'm glad I learned early, because it came in handy, both in school and out. This ability, however, goes beyond just avoiding nervousness while being pimped, as we'll talk about later.

So back to Dr. Steele. His questions would come at me fast and furious, and some I could answer. But for those I couldn't, he would not get the pleasure of seeing me sweat and fumble. I simply threw the ball back in his court with those three little words. With each day, I felt more and more comfortable. At one point, I was even smiling while confidently saying, "I didn't know", and could have sworn I caught him smiling back. But only for a second, and just as quickly as it appeared, it was gone, and he began teaching. I had broken him.

Chapter 27
Know-It-All

There is a constant pressure in medicine to know. Those with all of the answers are respected, revered. But as science advances, it becomes clear that there is too much information for any one person to master, even in a lifetime. The focus of medical education is slowly transforming into one in which you are not expected to know everything but simply know where to find the answers. Of course, there is a basic fund of knowledge every physician must know, but the days of memorizing entire text books are long gone. There are simply too many books.

But this transition is ongoing, and we are still in the earliest phases. The attendings in the hospital were mostly trained in the older style of medicine, where knowing was everything. This not only applies to medical facts, but also an expectation with patient care. There were some physicians who told medical students they should have their patient's information memorized, and should not use notes. A less aged physician would laugh at such an expectation. However, there is still a pressure to know answers, whether it be during pimping sessions or when asked about a patient's lab values. It creates an uncomfortable environment for providers, and quite frankly, an unsafe environment for patients. If an answer is unknown, there is always a pressure to say something. So, in response to a resident asking, "What was this patient's sodium value?", the medical student may vaguely remember, and although not definitively sure, state confidently, "137." Or, if they have no idea, say, "I think it's 137." The resident doesn't have time to remember which answers were prefaced with "I think" and takes responses at face value. Surely, the medical student will go back and double check later, but patient treatment may be delayed. One would think that when dealing with people's lives, there should be no ambiguity. Either you know, or you don't. Imagine a conversation between a pilot and air traffic control:

"JFK, this is flight 1296, what's our altitude?"

"Uh, 25,000 feet, I think."

That conversation simply does not happen in air traffic control, and medicine should be no exception. Hopefully, medicine will continue to progress towards a field where it is okay not to know all the answers, and our patients will actually benefit from our ignorance, so long as we can admit it.

Chapter 28

The Delivery

Perhaps nowhere in medical school do you get a better sense of the diversity in the social fabric of your community as you get in the OB/GYN department. During this rotation, the very personal aspects of people's lives are at the forefront, since factors such as living situation, sexual history, socioeconomic status, drug use, and family all play an important role in taking care of patients. For two months during our second year, we spent time with either the obstetrics service, in which we would take care of pregnant mothers, or in the gynecologic service, where we dealt with problems with the female reproductive system apart from child birth. The experience was particularly memorable, mostly due to a few very distinct cases.

My time on the obstetrics service started at a nearby hospital in Fayetteville, NC, hometown to Fort Bragg, a prominent army base. During the first few days on the service, we were called to evaluate a young woman that had gone into pre-term labor, and was in obvious pain and discomfort, much more than we typically see with child birth. The reason was that she had a cerclage in place. This is a device that, simply put, staples the end of your cervix together. It is used in women that have a history of multiple miscarriages with the thought that the miscarriage is due to the end of the cervix being too wide, and the uterus cannot hold the growing baby when the cervix remains open. This patient, however, had been very adamant about getting pregnant, and already had 11 miscarriages prior to this pregnancy! I could not believe what she must have gone through with the loss of each of those children. One would figure this was a woman that had been trying for a long time to get pregnant with her husband, and now was getting desperate as she was approaching middle age. But in fact, this patient was 22, single, with no job. She just simply wanted a child. Doing the math, if each of her pregnancies averaged 5 months, and if she was essentially pregnant all the time, she would have had to have started trying to get pregnant at 17. This was a conservative estimate, and chances are her attempts to conceive started years earlier.

So, the cerclage had been put in place early in the pregnancy, with hopes that if the problem was a loose cervix, the cerclage would keep things closed long enough to allow the child to be carried to term. Unfortunately, this woman was in active labor, and the baby was only about 22 weeks along. The lower limit of being able to sustain life outside of the womb is around 24 weeks. But her body was trying to squeeze out this child now, but the stitch in her cervix would not let the child out. The result was that her stitch was slowly tearing her cervix as the uterus continued to contract to get the child out. Not a good situation for the child or the mother.

Her pain and discomfort continued to worsen, and the obstetricians made every attempt possible to cut the cerclage, thereby opening her cervix and allowing her body to deliver the child. The child's chances of living would be slim given the extent of prematurity, but nothing would stop this woman's contractions. Her body wanted the baby out, and one way or another, her body would win. Unfortunately, her cervix had become so inflamed, they were unable to even see the cerclage, let alone cut it. So, the decision was made to put her under general anesthesia and deliver the child via C-section. A neonatal ICU doctor was called into the operating room to help with possibly resuscitating the baby if he was deemed mature enough to be able to sustain life. But when the C-section was performed, the infant that came out weighed a mere 400 grams, and was far from resembling a normal infant. The head seemed unusually large compared to a tiny, frail body. The infant's eye lids were still fused shut, another sign of extreme prematurity. The body was placed in an incubator while the neonatologist examined him, and it took less than 5 seconds for the physician to say this child was too premature to survive. Sadly, there was nothing that could be done for him, his body simply was not ready to be out of the womb. I watched him, as he lay there lifeless, and then suddenly, his chest contracted in a desperate attempt to get oxygen. He did this again every 30 seconds or so, but it was not long before even this movement stopped.

The mother had lost a great deal of blood during this time, but overall was stable. After the child was delivered, they were able to get to the cerclage, cut it, and remove it. She was taken back to the post-partum area and told of the news when she awoke. Her child had been wrapped up in blankets so that she could at least see him.

Sadly, he was already dead. However, she insisted on keeping him in her room for a while.

The next morning, I was saddened to find that she had kept the child next to her the entire night, refusing to accept the child she had so desperately wanted was once again not to be. It took some convincing to get her to finally let the child go, a true indication of just how badly she wanted to be a mother. But in my mind, I could only wonder what type of an environment such a child would have had to endure if in fact he had survived. This mother had little means for taking care of a child, and poor social support. Undoubtedly, it would have been a difficult life. And perhaps her multiple miscarriages were nature's way of saying that motherhood was not for her. However, I doubt she took the hint.

Sadly, there is no standard in society which determines who is worthy of having a child. Those types of standards only apply to more important things like owning a gun or adopting a pet. Take for example a woman I saw not long after this last case. She was about to deliver, so the obstetrics team was called to the case. She was a single woman, with no prenatal care, and a history of drug abuse during the pregnancy. She was alone at the delivery, with no apparent family support. Despite her transgressions, the fetus seemed to have done okay, and the delivery went smoothly. Out he came, and soon gave a vigorous cry. He was cleaned off quickly, and then wrapped up and handed to his mother, who he would meet face-to-face for the very first time. She took one look at him and said, "Oh my god, look at his nose, it's so big!" There was no motherly love, no smiles, no bonding, just simply a criticism, right from the start. Sure his nose may have been slightly generous in size, but nothing out of the norm, and otherwise, the child was beautiful. And to hear her say something negative about a newborn child just hurt me, probably because I see cases where parents try to do everything right during the pregnancy, take vitamins, go for regular check-ups, and not even drink caffeine, let alone even think about doing drugs, and the child is born with a horrendous heart or brain defect. And here she was, worried about the child's nose! When you see these infants, who are blank slates and full of potential, and they go home with these types of mothers, it just makes me sad. I know this child will fail in life, and due to no fault of his own, but because of his surroundings.

But I quickly learned that regardless of what we as physicians think is the right way to treat a child, either before or after the birth, society often has different ideas. A few weeks into the rotation, I was working in the clinic seeing expecting mothers for their routine prenatal visits.

That morning, I walked into a patient's room to start interviewing her and see how the pregnancy was going. Inside was a young woman, appeared to be in her mid 20's, well dressed, sitting comfortably. Her husband was with the army, and had been assigned to duty in another country, so she was there alone. The visit went smoothly, with little that was out of the ordinary. She was now in her second trimester, beginning to show. As I was wrapping up, I asked her if she had any other concerns before I brought the resident to come examine her.

"Well, there is something I was wondering about."

"Sure, what is it?" I asked.

And without any hesitation, she stated, "Well, I'm a stripper here at a local club, and my main trick is that I can climb the pole and do a split on the ceiling. Is it okay if I keep doing that while I'm pregnant?"

I wasn't quite sure where to start. Instead, I simply said I'd ask the resident. I didn't even want to start asking the hundreds of questions that came to mind. When I told the resident, she smiled slightly, but did not appear particularly phased. I'm sure she had heard it all. She simply went in, and told the patient that performing splits on the ceiling while pregnant was something she would advise against, and left it at that.

If this experience wasn't enough to make me realize that expecting mothers aren't always looking out for their unborn children, there was a couple that came in soon after our stripper friend that convinced me. They seemed like a very nice, polite couple, the type of couple I expected to see at these obstetrics appointments. The husband was very attentive to his wife, and asked insightful questions. But once again, near the end of the visit, he asked the question that made me angry.

"Is it okay if she continues to smoke marijuana during the pregnancy?"

He tried to defend his question by adding, "She has had a hard time with nausea, and marijuana really seems to be the only thing that will work for her." He conveniently left out the fact that it was also the only thing they had tried.

The resident had to answer based on the medical facts, "Up to this point, we do not have any definitive data that smoking marijuana may be detrimental to the fetus."

That was all they needed to hear, and I'm sure they were as happy as can be, ready to go home and smoke up with a clear conscience. And through the remainder of my rotation, I was amazed at the number of women that continued to smoke, drink alcohol, and even do drugs throughout the pregnancy.

But despite the saddening and frightening cases, the obstetrics rotation had its share of entertaining moments. Most distinctly was a case in which a woman was undergoing a simple procedure under anesthesia, and when she was ready for surgery, the surgeon noted a tattoo on the upper part of her thigh that said, "Mike's property." Let's hope Mike and her are still together, since that would be a tough one to explain to the next boyfriend. After seeing this tattoo, the surgeon began discussing some of the other tattoos he had seen in this region recently. One woman had a ruler tattooed onto the inside of her upper thigh, with a message underneath that said, "Can you measure up to this?" I'll let you decide what exactly she was measuring.

OBGYN also has the moment that is perhaps the most fulfilling throughout all of medical school – delivering your first baby. For me, this came late one night, after both myself and the resident had gone to our call rooms. The page came around 2AM from the nurse at the patient's bedside. Since labor takes so long, the doctors are called in at the last minute when the mother is ready to finally deliver, and sometimes even get there a bit late. So, I awoke out of my stupor, and stumbled my way to the patient's room. The resident got there soon after.

"This one's all yours."

I was ready. The process of childbirth is incredibly straightforward if things are going smoothly. After all, humans were delivering children long before we had obstetricians around. But when it's your first time delivering a baby, nothing is straightforward.

I took my position at the foot of the bed, and the nurse continued to coach the mother to push with each contraction. The baby's head was beginning to show with each push, coming out a bit further every time. My job was to hold the head, and as the baby was delivered, turn the head to the side and pull up and down on the head to allow the shoulders to come out. After the shoulders were through, I knew everything else would come shooting out quickly. The only thought running through my mind was, "Don't drop this baby!"

The head eventually made its way completely out, and I grabbed it with both hands, turned the head to the side, and pulled down to deliver one shoulder, then pulled up to deliver the other. Tons of green fluid rushed out as I did this, which means the child had already had its first bowel movement while still inside the uterus. As expected, the rest of the body came flying out soon afterwards, and I hung onto the infant's neck and legs as tight as possible without suffocating him. The resident helped cut the cord. He was a slippery little one, and despite my vigilance, there was still a moment where I felt him slipping, but I quickly readjusted my grip. The stimulation of the delivery was enough to get the newborn screaming, which is a sound every obstetrician loves to hear, because if the child isn't screaming, there is a problem. I quickly handed the child over to the mother. I was probably more excited about the delivery than she was. It was difficult to get back to bed after the excitement was over.

Overall, the OBGYN experience was a rollercoaster of emotions. Not everyone in society has the same priorities in life, which became quite clear during these two months. And despite the parts that were upsetting and disappointing, the moments of exhilaration were enough to make it all worthwhile.

Chapter 29

The Road

Meet John. John is a motivated high school student with high ambitions. He intends to get into the best college, and hopes to pick up a scholarship or two. All he has to do is dedicate all of his efforts to studying and participating in as many extra-curriculars as time will allow. He volunteers in the hospital and at the local food bank. When it comes to the SAT, he gets an early start and begins preparing when he is a freshman. All he has to do is sacrifice some fun now, and once he gets into college, he can finally relax.

Fast forward four years, and John is in college. All his hard work and weekend studying paid off. He is at one of the finest universities, and even earned himself a scholarship. He made it. But as he looks to the future, he decides that medicine is his calling. He's heard that getting into medical school is not easy. So he hits the books hard. He frequently passes up opportunities to go out with friends to sneak in a little extra study time. As a college junior, despite his busy schedule, he manages to meet a nice young girl who he is beginning to spend more time with. But the MCAT looms over his head, and his life is put totally on hold for a few months to completely focus on this exam. He and his girlfriend drift apart due to his focus on the test. "It's OK," he tells himself, there will be plenty of time for girls once he makes it through the MCAT and gets into medical school.

John does in fact make it into medical school. It took eight long years of hard work and commitment. But John does not have time to sit back and smell the roses, because after medical school looms residency. He intends to pursue a residency in internal medicine at one of the top hospitals, so he knows he has to buckle down. After all, he is competing with lots of very smart people across the country. Day after day of studying seem to fly by. Some of his medical school classmates decide to take salsa lessons to get a break from the daily grind, and John is invited to join them. But there is no time, and he decides to stay focused. Later in his medical school years he has to take Step 1, a board exam that residency programs use to rank applicants. For a few months, he lives and breathes from his study guide. In fact, there are a number of pages in this book marked by patches of drool where he fell asleep studying. He thinks back to how eerily similar this feels to studying for the SAT and MCAT. No worries though, this will all soon be over once he is a resident, because he will have made it, and can finally relax.

John is now an internal medicine resident, and finally, there are no more tests to study for. But he is working 80 hours each week, spending every fourth night in the hospital on call, with little time to breathe, let alone do the fun things he thought he'd finally have time for. Worse yet, John has decided he wants to pursue a cardiology fellowship, so tries to spend the small amount of time he has outside the hospital doing research so he can write the publications that will make him a better fellowship candidate.

You can see where this is going. John the cardiology fellow now has a greater level of responsibility in the hospital, and spends a large portion of his time trying to keep up with the latest literature in his field. But alas, after another three years as a fellow, John is finally done. He is finally a cardiologist. He is 33 years old, but he can finally relax, sit back, and enjoy life, right? Hardly, because he has an endless stream of patients that he needs to see to earn his keep in his private practice. And after every few years come those pesky recertification exams that he needs to pass to remain board certified.

So you see, it never ends...never! If you are sacrificing the things you love for your job, hoping there is only one more hoop to jump through, one more exam before you can relax, you will reach a sad realization when you are middle-aged and find that much of your youth has passed you by. Thankfully, I realized this early in life, and always made sure work did not get in the way of life. So take those weekend trips with friends, find a special someone in college, keeping playing that sport you love, and by all means, dance! The destination will never be worth it if you didn't enjoy the road.

Chapter 30
The End?

Four years soon came to an end. I found myself standing amongst my classmates, all of us garbed in our black and green graduation gowns. Our right hands were raised as we repeated the "Hippocratic Oath" in unison. This was our vow as doctors to "do no harm" and faithfully fulfill our new role. One by one, we walked across the stage, our parents beaming with pride from the audience. For the first time, we heard the new name which we would carry for the rest of our lives…

"Dr. Sujay Kansagra."

It felt a bit unreal. I had worked so hard for this, and yet still somehow felt unworthy of this new title. It carried a new sense of responsibility, along with a new sense of pride.

It was the last day many of us would ever see each other again. We would go off to our residencies all over the country and begin to specialize in our individual fields. But for now, we all celebrated together, with a common sense of accomplishment, and a sense of unity. We knew what each of us had gone through, something no one else would quite understand. The life, the death, the laughs, the tough times... we had been through it all together, and it was finally over. Soon, we would begin the next step. Our white coats would be longer, and our name tags would carry the letters "MD". With those two letters came a new world of expectations from others, where we could no longer hide in the comfort of, "I'm only a student." My stomach felt an uneasiness, and there was a sense of discomfort looming in the recesses of my mind. It was an all too familiar feeling, as I thought back to the start of medical school. It was the feeling of uncertainty and apprehension, mixed with anticipation. We would soon be pushed harder than ever before, in a world where the well-being of others would hang on our decisions. But the road ahead was also one in which we would develop into the doctors we had always dreamed we would be, and fine tune our knowledge in order to care for our patients. There would be a whole new set of challenges and experiences. But then again, it would undoubtedly bring new laughs, new friends, and new lessons.

So as we all said our final goodbyes and left the campus with our families, I knew this was by no means an ending, but the start of a brand new journey.

The Beginning

CPSIA information can be obtained at www.ICGtesting.com
Printed in the USA
LVOW101543251111

256468LV00001B/123/P